Teen Health Series

Pregnancy Information For Teens, Second Edition

Pregnancy Information For Teens,
Second Edition

Health Tips About Teen Pregnancy And Teen Parenting

Including Facts About Prenatal Care, Pregnancy Complications, Labor
And Delivery, Postpartum Care, Pregnancy-Related Lifestyle Concerns,
The Emotional And Legal Issues Of Teen Parenting, And More

Edited by Elizabeth Magill

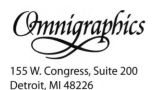

Omnigraphics

155 W. Congress, Suite 200
Detroit, MI 48226

Bibliographic Note

Because this page cannot legibly accommodate all the copyright notices, the Bibliographic Note portion of the Preface constitutes an extension of the copyright notice.

Edited by Elizabeth Magill

Teen Health Series

Karen Bellenir, *Managing Editor*
David A. Cooke, M.D., *Medical Consultant*
Elizabeth Collins, *Research and Permissions Coordinator*
Cherry Edwards, *Permissions Assistant*
EdIndex, *Services for Publishers, Indexers*

* * *

Omnigraphics, Inc.

Matthew P. Barbour, *Senior Vice President*
Kevin M. Hayes, *Operations Manager*

* * *

Peter E. Ruffner, *Publisher*
Copyright © 2012 Omnigraphics, Inc.
ISBN 978-0-7808-1220-8

Library of Congress Cataloging-in-Publication Data

Pregnancy information for teens : health tips about teen pregnancy and teen parenting including facts about prenatal care, pregnancy complications, labor and delivery, postpartum care, pregnancy-related lifestyle concerns, the emotional and legal issues of teen parenting, and more / edited by Elizabeth Magill. -- 2nd ed.
      p. cm.
   Summary: "Provides basic consumer information for teens about coping with an unplanned pregnancy including facts about staying healthy, preventing complications, preparing for childbirth, and facing the financial, legal, and emotional challenges of teen parenting. Includes index and resource information"-- Provided by publisher.
   Includes bibliographical references and index.
   ISBN 978-0-7808-1220-8 (hardcover : alk. paper) 1. Teenage parents. 2. Teenage pregnancy. I. Magill, Elizabeth, 1971-
   HQ759.64.P72 2012
   618.200835--dc23
                                                                                2011042323

Table of Contents

Part Four: High-Risk Pregnancies And Pregnancy Complications

Part Five: Childbirth

Part Six: Your Newborn

Part Seven: Teen Parenting Problems And Solutions

Preface

About This Book

According to recent data from the Centers for Disease Control and Prevention, the U.S. teenage birth rate reached a historic low in 2009, at 39.1 births per 1,000 women aged 15–19. Despite this encouraging news, the U.S. teenage birth rate retained its distinction of being the highest among industrialized countries, emphasizing the nation's need for continued efforts at helping young women avoid unplanned pregnancies.

Teenage pregnancy is associated with diverse risks. Teenage mothers have a higher risk of preterm labor and delivery, anemia, preeclampsia, and other pregnancy complications. Babies born to teenage mothers have higher risks for low birthweight, serious health problems, and even death. Some pregnant teens may lack access to proper nutrition or may participate in risky activities, such as smoking, drinking alcohol, and taking drugs, which can have a negative effect on maternal and fetal health. In addition to such physical concerns, teenage mothers—and fathers—face other social and emotional risks, including negotiating relationships with each other and with their parents. Furthermore, they are less likely than their peers to complete their education and find well-paying jobs.

Pregnancy Information For Teens, Second Edition discusses the bewildering array of choices to be made and the obstacles to be overcome when a young woman faces an unplanned pregnancy. It includes facts about abortion, adoption, prenatal care, nutrition, fetal development, and preparing for labor and delivery. For teens choosing to parent their infants, it offers information on how to care for a newborn, locate and pay for child care, and receive child support. It discusses the importance of completing an education and describes the public assistance programs that are available, including assistance with health insurance and living arrangements. An end section provides information about sources of help and directories of additional resources.

How To Use This Book

This book is divided into parts and chapters. Parts focus on broad areas of interest; chapters are devoted to single topics within a part.

Part One: Understanding The Problem Of Teen Pregnancy discusses the serious consequences teen pregnancy has on the mother, the child, and on society. It also presents information on two models for pregnancy prevention (abstinence-only and comprehensive sexuality education) and discusses the recent changes in federal sexual education policy. There is also a chapter on teen pregnancy and the media that explores the impact of recent TV shows on teens' perceptions of pregnancy and parenting.

Part Two: If You Think You're Pregnant provides information on the signs and symptoms of pregnancy and facts about pregnancy tests. After a pregnancy is confirmed, pregnant teens must make a difficult choice—abortion, adoption, or parenting. Individual chapters within this part discuss each of these alternatives.

Part Three: Staying Healthy During Your Pregnancy talks about what a pregnant teen must do—and not do—in order to have a healthy pregnancy. It includes information on prenatal care, tests and procedures, sleep, nutrition, and exercise. It also explains why alcohol, tobacco, illegal drugs, and some other substances must be avoided during pregnancy. Finally, there is a chapter on protecting yourself and getting help if you are in an abusive relationship while pregnant.

Part Four: High-Risk Pregnancies And Pregnancy Complications discusses various conditions that may be present before pregnancy that increase the risk of complications, such as asthma and diabetes. It also discusses conditions that can arise during pregnancy, such as gestational diabetes and preeclampsia.

Part Five: Childbirth describes the many ways to prepare for childbirth, such as birthing classes, birth plans, and choosing a birth location. It also presents information on labor, birth, and recovery.

Part Six: Your Newborn gives teen mothers important information about what happens during a newborn's first hours of life, including health assessments and screening tests. It also answers questions about breastfeeding and gives tips on taking care of a baby at home.

Part Seven: Teen Parenting Problems And Solutions discusses the many unique challenges teen parents face, including child care options, finding a place to live, and finishing school. Important facts about child custody, child care, and health insurance are presented along with public assistance options for teen parents, including supplemental nutrition and vaccine programs. Finally, there is a chapter about the rights and responsibilities of teen fathers.

Part Eight: If You Need More Information includes directories of teen pregnancy resources, assistance for low-income pregnant women, and education resources for teen parents.

Bibliographic Note

This volume contains documents and excerpts from publications issued by the following government agencies: Centers for Disease Control and Prevention (CDC); National Institute of Child Health and Human Development (NICHD); National Institute of Diabetes and Digestive and Kidney Diseases (NIDDK); U.S. Department of Agriculture (USDA); U.S. Department of Health and Human Services; U.S. Department of Housing and Urban Development (HUD); and the U.S. Food and Drug Administration (FDA).

In addition, this volume contains copyrighted documents and articles produced by the following organizations: About, Inc; A.D.A.M., Inc; American College of Allergy, Asthma and Immunology; American Pregnancy Association; Guttmacher Institute; March of Dimes Birth Defects Foundation; Merck & Co, Inc; National Association of Child Care Resource & Referral Agencies (NACCRRA); The National Campaign to Prevent Teen Pregnancy; The Nemours Foundation; Pennsylvania Bar Association; Planned Parenthood Federation of America, Inc; Preeclampsia Foundation; Public Counsel; Sexuality Information and Education Council of the United States (SIECUS); South Eastern Centre Against Sexual Assault (SECASA); and the University of North Carolina Chapel Hill School of Government

The photograph on the front cover is from E. Dygas/Getty Images.

Full citation information is provided on the first page of each chapter. Every effort has been made to secure all necessary rights to reprint the copyrighted material. If any omissions have been made, please contact Omnigraphics to make corrections for future editions.

Acknowledgements

In addition to the organizations listed above, special thanks are due to Liz Collins, research and permissions coordinator; Karen Bellenir, managing editor; Lisa Bakewell, verification assistant; and WhimsyInk, prepress services provider.

About the *Teen Health Series*

At the request of librarians serving today's young adults, the *Teen Health Series* was developed as a specially focused set of volumes within Omnigraphics' *Health Reference Series*. Each volume deals comprehensively with a topic selected according to the needs and interests of people in middle school and high school.

Teens seeking preventive guidance, information about disease warning signs, medical statistics, and risk factors for health problems will find answers to their questions in the *Teen*

Health Series. The *Series*, however, is not intended to serve as a tool for diagnosing illness, in prescribing treatments, or as a substitute for the physician/patient relationship. All people concerned about medical symptoms or the possibility of disease are encouraged to seek professional care from an appropriate health care provider.

If there is a topic you would like to see addressed in a future volume of the *Teen Health Series*, please write to:

Editor
Teen Health Series
Omnigraphics, Inc.
155 W. Congress, Suite 200
Detroit, MI 48226

A Note about Spelling and Style

Teen Health Series editors use *Stedman's Medical Dictionary* as an authority for questions related to the spelling of medical terms and the *Chicago Manual of Style* for questions related to grammatical structures, punctuation, and other editorial concerns. Consistent adherence is not always possible, however, because the individual volumes within the *Series* include many documents from a wide variety of different producers and copyright holders, and the editor's primary goal is to present material from each source as accurately as is possible following the terms specified by each document's producer. This sometimes means that information in different chapters or sections may follow other guidelines and alternate spelling authorities. For example, occasionally a copyright holder may require that eponymous terms be shown in possessive forms (Crohn's disease *vs.* Crohn disease) or that British spelling norms be retained (leukaemia *vs.* leukemia).

Locating Information within the *Teen Health Series*

The *Teen Health Series* contains a wealth of information about a wide variety of medical topics. As the *Series* continues to grow in size and scope, locating the precise information needed by a specific student may become more challenging. To address this concern, information about books within the *Teen Health Series* is included in *A Contents Guide to the Health Reference Series*. The *Contents Guide* presents an extensive list of more than 16,000 diseases, treatments, and other topics of general interest compiled from the Tables of Contents and major index headings from the books of the *Teen Health Series* and *Health Reference Series*. To access *A Contents Guide to the Health Reference Series*, visit www.healthreferenceseries.com.

Our Advisory Board

We would like to thank the following advisory board members for providing guidance to the development of this *Series*:

Dr. Lynda Baker, Associate Professor of Library and Information Science, Wayne State University, Detroit, MI

Nancy Bulgarelli, William Beaumont Hospital Library, Royal Oak, MI

Karen Imarisio, Bloomfield Township Public Library, Bloomfield Township, MI

Karen Morgan, Mardigian Library, University of Michigan-Dearborn, Dearborn, MI

Rosemary Orlando, St. Clair Shores Public Library, St. Clair Shores, MI

Medical Consultant

Medical consultation services are provided to the *Teen Health Series* editors by David A. Cooke, M.D. Dr. Cooke is a graduate of Brandeis University, and he received his M.D. degree from the University of Michigan. He completed residency training at the University of Wisconsin Hospital and Clinics. He is board-certified in internal medicine. Dr. Cooke currently works as part of the University of Michigan Health System and practices in Ann Arbor, MI. In his free time, he enjoys writing, science fiction, and spending time with his family.

Part One
Understanding The Problem Of Teen Pregnancy

Chapter 1

The Risks Of Teenage Pregnancy

Teenage birth rates in the United States are high, exceeding those in most developed countries.

High teen birth rates are an important concern because teen mothers and their babies face increased risks to their health, and their opportunities to build a future are diminished.

Here are some important facts about teen pregnancy:

- More than 10 percent of all U.S. births in 2006 were to mothers under age 20. Most teenage births (about 67 percent) are to girls ages 18 and 19.

- The pregnancy rate for teenagers fell 40 percent between 1990 and 2005 (from 116.8 to 70.6 per 1,000). However, in 2005, about 725,000 teens ages 15 to 19 became pregnant, and about 415,000 gave birth.

- About three in 10 teenage girls become pregnant at least once before age 20.

- The teenage birth rate increased in 2006 and 2007. Between 2005 and 2007, the rate rose five percent (from 41 to 42.5 per 1,000 women). This increase follows a 14-year decline between 1991 and 2005, when the rate fell by one-third (from 62 to 41 per 1,000 women). In 2007, about four in 100 teenage girls had a baby.

- About one in four teen mothers under age 18 have a second baby within two years after the birth of their first baby.

- Teen mothers are more likely than mothers over age 20 to give birth prematurely (before 37 completed weeks of pregnancy). Between 2003 and 2005, preterm birth rates

About This Chapter: Information in this chapter is from "Teenage pregnancy," © 2009 March of Dimes Birth Defects Foundation. All rights reserved. For additional information, contact the March of Dimes at their website www.marchofdimes.com.

averaged 14.5 percent for women under age 20 compared to 11.9 percent for women ages 20 to 29. Babies born prematurely face an increased risk of newborn health problems, long-term disabilities, and even death.

How does a teen mother's health affect her baby?

Some teens may need to change their lifestyle to improve their chances of having a healthy baby. Eating unhealthy foods, smoking, drinking alcohol, and taking drugs can increase the risk that a baby will be born with health problems, such as low birthweight (less than 5 ½ pounds).

Teens are more likely than women over age 25 to smoke during pregnancy. In 2004, 17 percent of pregnant teens ages 15 to 19 smoked, compared to 10 percent of pregnant women ages 25 to 34. Babies of women who smoke during pregnancy are at increased risk for premature birth, low birthweight, and sudden infant death syndrome (SIDS). Women who smoke during pregnancy also have an increased risk for pregnancy complications, including placental problems.

Teens are least likely of all maternal age groups to get early and regular prenatal care. From 2000 to 2002, an average 7.1 percent of mothers under age 20 received late or no prenatal care, compared to 3.7 percent for all ages.

Of 19 million new cases of sexually transmitted infections (STIs) reported each year, more than nine million affect young people ages 15 to 24. These STIs include:

- Chlamydia, which can cause sterility in the affected individual and eye infections and pneumonia in the newborn.

- Syphilis, which can cause blindness, maternal death, and infant death.

- Human immunodeficiency virus (HIV), the virus that causes acquired immune deficiency syndrome (AIDS). Treatment during pregnancy greatly reduces the risk of an infected mother passing HIV to her baby.

It's A Fact!

A teenage mother is at greater risk than women over age 20 for pregnancy complications, such as premature labor, anemia, and high blood pressure. These risks are even greater for teens who are under 15 years old.

What are the health risks to babies of teen mothers?

A baby born to a teenage mother is at higher risk than a baby born to an older mother for premature birth, low birthweight, other serious health problems, and death.

Babies of teenage mothers are more likely to die in the first year of life than babies of women in their twenties and thirties. The risk is highest for babies of mothers under age 15. In 2005, 16.4 out of every 1,000 babies of women under age 15 died, compared to 6.8 per 1,000 for babies of women of all ages.

Teenage mothers are more likely to have a low-birthweight baby. Most low-birthweight babies are born prematurely. The earlier a baby is born, the less she is likely to weigh. In 2006, 10 percent of mothers ages 15 to 19 had a low-birthweight baby, compared to 8.3 percent for mothers of all ages. The risk is higher for younger mothers:

- 11.7 percent of 15-year-old mothers had a low-birthweight baby in 2006; 18,403 babies were born to girls this age, with 2,153 of low birthweight.

- 9.5 percent of 19-year-old mothers had a low-birthweight baby in 2006; 172,999 babies were born to these women, with 16,362 of low birthweight.

Babies who are premature and low birthweight may have organs that are not fully developed. This can lead to breathing problems, such as respiratory distress syndrome, bleeding in the brain, vision loss, and serious intestinal problems.

Very low-birthweight babies (less than 3⅓ pounds) are more than 100 times as likely to die, and moderately low-birthweight babies (between 3⅓ and 5½ pounds) are more than five times as likely to die in their first year of life than normal-weight babies.

What are other consequences of teenage pregnancy?

Life may be difficult for a teenage mother and her child. Teen mothers are more likely to drop out of high school than girls who delay childbearing. Only 40 percent of teenagers who have children before age 18 go on to graduate from high school, compared to 75 percent of teens from similar social and economic backgrounds who do not give birth until ages 20 or 21.

With her education cut short, a teenage mother may lack job skills, making it hard for her to find and keep a job. A teenage mother may become financially dependent on her family or on public assistance. Teen mothers are more likely to live in poverty than women who delay childbearing, and more than 75 percent of all unmarried teen mothers go on welfare within five years of the birth of their first child.

About 64 percent of children born to an unmarried teenage high-school dropout live in poverty, compared to seven percent of children born to women over age 20 who are married and high school graduates. A child born to a teenage mother is 50 percent more likely to repeat a grade in school and is more likely to perform poorly on standardized tests and drop out before finishing high school.

What recommendations does the March of Dimes make to guide teenage girls?

Because of the risks involved in teen pregnancy to both mother and child, the March of Dimes strongly urges teenage girls to delay childbearing. The March of Dimes also recommends that anyone who could become pregnant eat a healthy diet, achieve a healthy weight, and quit smoking.

The March of Dimes further recommends that all women, including teens, who could become pregnant, take a multivitamin containing folic acid every day for the teen's own health and to reduce the risk of having a baby with birth defects of the brain and spinal cord, should they become pregnant.

Teens who already are pregnant can improve their chances of having a healthy baby by:

- Getting early and regular prenatal care from a health care provider or clinic.

- Eating a nutritious and balanced diet.

- Stopping smoking and avoiding secondhand smoke. Smoking increases the risk for low birthweight, premature birth, pregnancy complications, and sudden infant death syndrome (SIDS).

- Stopping drinking alcohol and/or using illicit drugs. Alcohol and drug use limit fetal growth and can cause birth defects.

- Avoiding all prescription and over-the-counter drugs (including herbal preparations), unless recommended by a health care provider who is aware of the pregnancy.

Chapter 2

Recent Teen Pregnancy Statistics

Teenage childbearing has been the subject of long-standing concern among the public and policy makers. Teenagers who give birth are much more likely to deliver a low birthweight or preterm infant than older women, and their babies are at elevated risk of dying in infancy. The annual public costs associated with teen childbearing have been estimated at $9.1 billion. The U.S. teen birth rate fell by more than one-third from 1991 through 2005, but then increased by five percent over two consecutive years. Data for 2008 and 2009, however, indicate that the long-term downward trend has resumed. Although the recent declines have been widespread by age, race and ethnicity, and state, large disparities nevertheless persist in these characteristics. The most current data available from the National Vital Statistics System are used to illustrate trends and variations through 2009.

Teen Birth Rate In 2009

- The U.S. birth rate for teenagers in 2009 was the lowest it has ever been in the nearly 70 years for which national data are available. The rate was 39.1 births per 1,000 females aged 15–19 years, 37 percent below the 1991 rate (61.8), the most recent peak.

- The teenage birth rate in 2009 was 59 percent lower than the historic high reached in 1957 (96.3).

- The number of births to teenagers aged 15–19 in 2009 fell to 409,840, the fewest since 1946, and 36 percent fewer than in 1970 (644,708), the historic high point.

About This Chapter: Information in this chapter is from Ventura SJ, Hamilton BE. "U.S. teenage birth rate resumes decline," NCHS data brief, no 58. Hyattsville, MD: National Center for Health Statistics. 2011.

Key Findings

- The teenage birth rate declined 8% in the United States from 2007 through 2009, reaching a historic low at 39.1 births per 1,000 teens aged 15–19 years.

- Rates fell significantly for teenagers in all age groups and for all racial and ethnic groups.

- Teenage birth rates for each age group and for nearly all race and Hispanic origin groups in 2009 were at the lowest levels ever reported in the United States.

- Birth rates for teens aged 15–17 dropped in 31 states from 2007 through 2009; rates for older teenagers aged 18–19 declined significantly in 45 states during this period.

Recent Declines For Younger And Older Teenagers

- The birth rate for young teenagers aged 15–17 fell 7% in 2009 from 2008, the largest single-year drop since 2000–2001. The 2009 rate (20.1 per 1,000), a historic low, was 48 percent lower than in 1991 (38.6 per 1,000).

- The birth rate for older teenagers aged 18–19 fell 6% from 2008 through 2009, the largest single-year decline since 1971–1972. The 2009 rate, also a historic low at 66.2 per 1,000, was 30 percent lower than in 1991 (94.0).

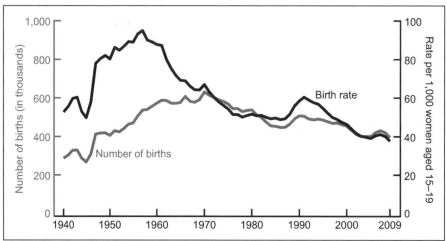

NOTES: Data for 2009 are preliminary. Data table for Figure 2.1 is available from:
http://www.cdc.gov/nchs/data/databriefs/db58_tables.pdf#1.
SOURCE: CDC/NCHS, National Vital Statistics System.

Figure 2.1. Number of births and birth rates for teenagers aged 15–19: United States, 1940–2009

- Births and birth rates for the youngest teenagers, under age 15, have also declined over the last half century. The 2009 birth rate for females aged 10–14 was 0.5 births per 1,000, the lowest ever reported and two-thirds lower than in 1990 (1.4). Moreover, the number of babies born to this age group has fallen to the fewest in nearly 60 years, to 5,030 in 2009.

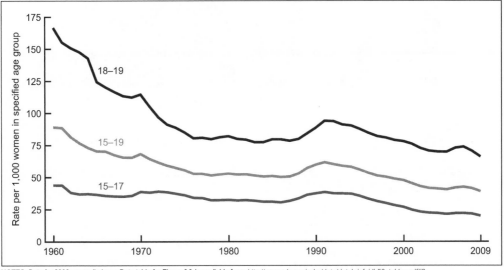

NOTES: Data for 2009 are preliminary. Data table for Figure 2.2 is available from: http://www.cdc.gov/nchs/data/databriefs/db58_tables.pdf#2.
SOURCE: CDC/NCHS, National Vital Statistics System.

Figure 2.2. Birth rates for teenagers, by age: United States, 1960–2009

Falling Birth Rates For Teenagers Aged 15–17

- Birth rates for white and black non-Hispanic teenagers and Asian or Pacific Islander (API) teenagers aged 15–17 dropped 53% to 63% from 1991 through 2009.

- Although the birth rate for Hispanic teenagers declined more slowly overall from 1991 through 2009, the decline in the rate from 2008 to 2009 (41.0 per 1,000) was the largest of all race and ethnicity groups (by 11%).

- Further, the rate for Hispanic teenagers in 2009 was the lowest ever recorded in the two decades for which rates are available for this group.

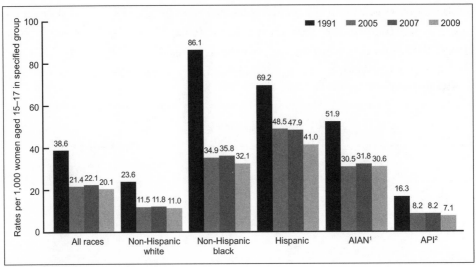

¹American Indian or Alaska Native.
²Asian or Pacific Islander.
NOTES: Data for 2009 are preliminary. Data table for Figure 2.3 is available from: http://www.cdc.gov/nchs/data/databriefs/db58_tables.pdf#3.
SOURCE: CDC/NCHS, National Vital Statistics System.

Figure 2.3. Birth rates for teenagers aged 15–17, by race and Hispanic origin: United States, 1991, 2005, 2007, and 2009

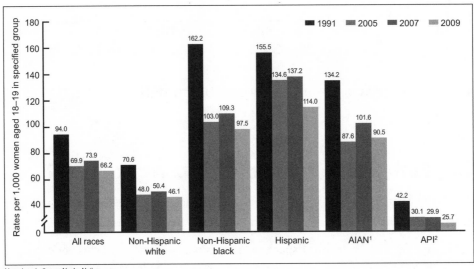

¹American Indian or Alaska Native.
²Asian or Pacific Islander.
NOTES: Data for 2009 are preliminary. Data table for Figure 2.4 is available from: http://www.cdc.gov/nchs/data/databriefs/db58_tables.pdf#4.
SOURCE: CDC/NCHS, National Vital Statistics System.

Figure 2.4. Birth rates for teenagers aged 18–19, by race and Hispanic origin: United States, 1991, 2005, 2007, and 2009

Falling Birth Rates For Teenagers Aged 18–19

- Birth rates overall and by race and ethnicity are consistently higher for ages 18–19 than for ages 15–17. Although the downward trend for both age groups has been similar, long-term declines were smaller for older teenagers.

- From 1991 through 2009, rates for all racial and ethnic groups for ages 18–19 dropped by 27% to 40%. Single-year declines for all groups from 2008 to 2009 ranged from 5% to 10%.

- Birth rates in 2009 for non-Hispanic white (46.1 per 1,000), non-Hispanic black (97.5), and API teenagers (25.7) were the lowest ever reported for these groups. Similarly, the 2009 rate for Hispanic teenagers aged 18–19 was a record low (114.0).

Falling Birth Rates For Young Teenagers In Most States During 2007–2009

- Birth rates for teenagers aged 15–17 fell significantly in most areas of the country from 2007 through 2009, the most recent period of decline for teen birth rates.

- The largest declines were in the intermountain West and southeast areas of the United States. The decline in rates ranged from 5% for Ohio and Indiana to 20% for Arizona.

- The rate increased significantly for only one state from 2007 through 2009, West Virginia, by 17%.

- Birth rates for older teenagers aged 18–19 fell in 45 states from 2007 through 2009.

- Birth rates fell for ages 18–19 from 2007 through 2009 in the majority of states. The largest declines were reported for the intermountain West and northern New England states.

- The range of decline was from 5% for New York, Louisiana, and New Mexico to 27% for New Hampshire and Vermont.

The U.S. teenage birth rate reached a historic low in 2009, at 39.1 births per 1,000 women aged 15–19. While the U.S. teenage birth rate fell 37 percent from 1991 through 2009, it still remains the highest among industrialized countries. Rates in the United States fell from 2007 through 2009 by age subgroup, race and Hispanic origin, and state. The recent trend marks a resumption of the long-term decline in teenage childbearing that started in 1991. Previous studies have suggested that these declines reflected the impact of strong teenage pregnancy prevention messages that accompanied a variety of public and private efforts to focus teenagers' attention on the importance of avoiding pregnancy. Data from several cycles of the National

Survey of Family Growth (NSFG) conducted by the Centers for Disease Control and Prevention's National Center for Health Statistics (CDC/NCHS) showed that teen sexual activity declined or leveled off in the 1990s through the mid-2000s, and that contraceptive use increased or stabilized. Data from the 2006–2010 NSFG, forthcoming in 2011, may be helpful in identifying the factors associated with the declines in teenage birth rates.

Data Sources And Methods

This report contains data from the Natality Data File, National Vital Statistics System. The vital statistics natality file includes information for all births occurring in the United States. The natality files, which cover a wide range of maternal and infant demographic and health characteristics, are available from the NCHS website: http://www.cdc.gov/nchs/data_access/VitalStatsOnline.htm. Data may also be accessed using the interactive data access tool VitalStats, available from: http://www.cdc.gov/nchs/VitalStats.htm.

State-specific birth rates for teenagers for 2009 are based on preliminary birth data. Information on the 2009 data is available elsewhere. Population data for computing birth rates were provided by the U.S. Census Bureau. Rates by state shown here may differ from rates computed on the basis of other population estimates.

What's It Mean?

Teenage Birth Rate: The number of births to women aged 15–19 (or teenage subgroup) per 1,000 women aged 15–19 (or teenage subgroup).

Chapter 3

When Pregnancy Is A Result Of Abuse

Domestic violence is when one person in a relationship purposely hurts another person physically or emotionally. Domestic violence is also called intimate partner violence because it often is caused by a husband, ex-husband, boyfriend, or ex-boyfriend. Women also can be abusers.

People of all races, education levels, and ages experience domestic abuse. In the United States, more than five million women are abused by an intimate partner each year.

Domestic violence includes behaviors such as these:

- Physical abuse like hitting, shoving, kicking, biting, or throwing things
- Emotional abuse like yelling, controlling what you do, or threatening to cause serious problems for you
- Sexual abuse like forcing you to do something sexual you don't want to do

Here are some key points about domestic and intimate partner violence:

- **If you are in immediate danger, you can call 911.** It is possible for the police to arrest an abuser and to escort you and your children to a safe place.
- **Often, abuse starts as emotional abuse and then becomes physical later.** It's important to get help early.
- **Sometimes it is hard to know if you are being abused.** You can learn more about signs of abuse at http://www.womenshealth.gov/violence-against-women/am-i-being-abused/index.cfm.

About This Chapter: Information in this chapter is from the following publications of the U.S. Department of Health and Human Services: "Domestic and intimate partner violence," May 2011; "Staying healthy and safe," September 2010.

- **Your partner may try to make you feel like the abuse is your fault.** Remember that you cannot make someone mistreat you. The abuser is responsible for his or her behavior. Abuse can be a way for your partner to try to have control over you.

- **Violence can cause serious physical and emotional problems, including depression and post-traumatic stress disorder.** It's important to try to take care of your health. And if you are using drugs or alcohol to cope with abuse, get help.

- **There probably will be times when your partner is very kind.** Unfortunately, abusers often begin the mistreatment again after these periods of calm. In fact, over time, abuse often gets worse, not better. Even if your partner promises to stop the abuse, make sure to learn about hotlines and other ways to get help for abuse.

- **An abusive partner needs to get help from a mental health professional.** But even if he or she gets help, the abuse may not stop.

Being hurt by someone close to you is awful. Reach out for support from family, friends, and community organizations.

Abuse And Pregnancy

It's hard to be excited about the new life growing inside of you if you're afraid of your partner. Abuse from a partner can begin or increase during pregnancy and can harm you and your unborn baby. Women who are abused often don't get the prenatal care their babies need. Abuse from a partner also can lead to preterm birth and low birthweight babies, stillbirth and newborn death, and homicide. If you are abused, you might turn to alcohol, cigarettes, or drugs to help you cope. This can be even more harmful to you and your baby.

You may think that a new baby will change your situation for the better. But the cycle of abuse is complex, and a baby introduces new stress to people and relationships. Now is a good

---

Quick Tip

Sometimes, abuse begins when you are pregnant. Abuse can cause serious health problems for a baby even before it is born. Also, some men try to stop their partners from using birth control. Talk to your doctor about protecting your health and about birth control that you can use without your partner knowing.

Source: From "Domestic and intimate partner violence," a publication of the U.S. Department of Health and Human Services, May 2011.

Emotional Impact

For many women the emotional and psychological impact of rape creates post traumatic stress disorder (PTSD), and symptoms are often exacerbated when the victim/survivor gives birth. Pregnancy following rape is more likely to lead to inner conflicts for women about deciding whether to keep the child or not. Long term effects may include depression, as many women may blame themselves, and experience feelings of shame and guilt that can then project onto their growing child.

Grief issues surrounding pregnancy following rape may arise in relation to the woman's decision about whether to keep her child or to have a termination.

With the support of family and friends, many women are able to overcome the psychological and emotional trauma and maintain a healthy relationship with their child.

Source: Excerpted from "Pregnancy Following Rape," © 2009 South Eastern Centre Against Sexual Assault (SECASA) (www.secasa.com.au). Reprinted with permission.

time to think about your safety and the safety and wellbeing of your baby. About 50 percent of men who abuse their wives also abuse their children. Think about the home environment you want for your baby. Studies show that children who witness or experience violence at home may have long-term physical, emotional, and social problems. They are also more likely to experience or commit violence themselves in the future.

Prenatal exams offer a good chance to reach out for help. It's possible to take control and leave an abusive partner. But for your and your baby's safety, talk to your doctor first. Let motherhood prompt you to take action now.

If you're a victim of abuse or violence at the hands of someone you know or love, or you are recovering from an assault by a stranger, you and your baby can get immediate help and support.

The National Domestic Violence Hotline External Website Policy can be reached 24 hours a day, seven days a week at 800-799-SAFE (7233) and 800-787-3224 (TTY). Spanish speakers are available. When you call, you will first hear a recording and may have to hold. Hotline staff offer crisis intervention and referrals. If requested, they connect women to shelters and can send out written information.

The National Sexual Assault Hotline External Website Policy can be reached 24 hours a day, seven days a week at 800-656-4673. When you call, you will hear a menu and can choose number one to talk to a counselor. You will then be connected to a counselor in your area who can help you. You can also visit the National Sexual Assault Online Hotline External Website Policy.

Chapter 4

Preventing Teen Pregnancy

New White House Initiative Overhauls U.S. Teen Pregnancy Prevention Efforts

Requires Programs To Be Effective, Age-Appropriate, And Medically Accurate, But Key Details Remain Unresolved

The $114.5 million teen pregnancy prevention initiative signed into law by President Obama in December 2009 marks a major turning point in U.S. sex education policy, according to a new analysis published in the Winter 2010 issue of the Guttmacher Policy Review. The initiative replaces many of the most rigid and ineffective abstinence-only programs, which by law were required to have nonmarital abstinence promotion as their "exclusive purpose" and were prohibited from discussing the benefits of contraception.

However, this welcome course correction is tempered somewhat by the late-breaking news that congressional leaders appear to have agreed—per a provision in the final version of the health care reform legislation moving through Congress—to resuscitate the Title V abstinence-only program for five years (see "About The Title V Program" later in this chapter for more information on this program).

About This Chapter: Information in this chapter is from the Guttmacher Institute, "New White House Initiative Overhauls U.S. Teen Pregnancy Prevention Efforts," news release, New York: Guttmacher, March 22, 2010, http://www.guttmacher.org/media/nr/2010/03/22/index.html, accessed August 26, 2011. Additional text under the heading "Teen Pregnancy In The United States" is from "Preventing Teen Pregnancy 2010–2015," Centers for Disease Control and Prevention, 2010.

In sharp contrast to the failed abstinence-only policies of the past, the new approach championed by the White House will focus on programs that have demonstrated their effectiveness, and all funded programs will be required to be age-appropriate and medically accurate.

"The administration's teen pregnancy prevention initiative is an important victory for evidence-based policymaking," says Heather Boonstra, author of the new analysis. "The next step is critical—finalizing implementation details and regulations that determine which specific programs get funded."

The initiative will be administered by a newly created Office of Adolescent Health within the Department of Health and Human Services (DHHS), working in cooperation with the Administration for Children and Families, the Centers for Disease Control and Prevention, and other relevant DHHS agencies. According to Boonstra, officials will need to determine which programs meet the following funding criteria laid out in the legislation:

- **Effective Or Promising:** A large body of evidence shows that more comprehensive approaches—those that encourage abstinence, but also contraceptive use for young people who are having sex—can be effective. But rigid, moralistic abstinence-only programs of the type promoted under previous federal policy have not been found to be effective (which is not to say that no intervention focusing only on abstinence can ever work for any population under any circumstances).

- **Age-Appropriate:** Because adolescence is a time of rapid change, sex education interventions must adapt as young people change. Emphasizing only abstinence may be appropriate for lower grade levels, when very few students are having sex; however, once a significant proportion of students are sexually active, programs should progressively include more information about contraceptives and less about abstinence.

- **Medically Accurate:** Strict requirements for medical accuracy should apply to any programs funded under the initiative. The withholding of relevant information should be considered, per se, inaccurate—and denigration of condoms or contraceptives, directly or indirectly, preemptively prohibited.

"While it is deeply disappointing that it appears likely that the Title V abstinence-only program will survive in some form, we nevertheless have entered a new era in U.S. sex education policy—and not a moment too soon," says Boonstra. "For the first time in more than a decade, the nation's teen pregnancy rate rose in 2006, by 3%—and the increase coincided with the major funding boosts for abstinence-only programs under the Bush administration. Rigid abstinence-only programs truly are a failed experiment and Congress needs to stop funding them altogether."

Following a steep decline in the 1990s and a flattening out in the early 2000s, teen pregnancy rates increased among all ethnic and racial groups between 2005 and 2006. Earlier research had documented that the significant drop in teen pregnancy rates in the 1990s overwhelmingly had been the result of more and better use of contraceptives among sexually active teens. However, this decline started to stall out in the early 2000s, at the same time that abstinence-only programs became more widespread, teens were receiving less information about contraception in schools and their use of contraceptives was declining.

About The Title V Program

The Title V abstinence-only program, which appears to have been have resuscitated in the final version of the health care reform legislation moving through Congress, would offer $50 million in grants to the states annually for five years. Programs funded under Title V must conform to a highly restrictive, eight-point definition—a policy that flies in the face of strong evidence that such rigid, moralistic programs do not work. By the time the Title V abstinence-only program expired in June 2009, roughly half the states had declined to apply for funding under the program, in large part because these programs have proven ineffective.

At the same time, health care reform—if enacted—would not only fund Title V, but would also provide $75 million per year over five years for a new "personal responsibility education program," most of which would go toward programs that educate adolescents about both abstinence and contraception, and are evidence-based, medically accurate, and age appropriate. Going forward, this means that a total of about $190 million in federal funding would be made available for evidence-based programs ($114.5 million from the new teen pregnancy prevention initiative and $75 million from health care reform), while $50 million would be offered for rigid abstinence-only programs.

Teen Pregnancy In The United States

In 2008, 435,000 live births occurred to mothers aged 15–19 years, a birth rate of 41.5 per 1,000 women in this age group. Nearly two-thirds of births to mothers younger than age 18 and more than half among mothers aged 18–19 years are unintended. The U.S. teen pregnancy and birth, sexually transmitted diseases (STDs), and abortion rates are substantially higher than those of other western industrialized nations.

The Importance Of Prevention

Teen pregnancy and childbearing bring substantial social and economic costs through immediate and long-term impacts on teen parents and their children.

- Teen pregnancy accounts for more than $9 billion per year in costs to U.S. taxpayers for increased health care and foster care, increased incarceration rates among children of teen parents, and lost tax revenue because of lower educational attainment and income among teen mothers.

- Pregnancy and birth are significant contributors to high school dropout rates among girls. Only about 50% of teen mothers receive a high school diploma by age 22, versus nearly 90% of women who had not given birth during adolescence.

- The children of teenage mothers are more likely to have lower school achievement and drop out of high school, have more health problems, be incarcerated at some time during adolescence, give birth as a teenager, and face unemployment as a young adult.

These effects remain for the teen mother and her child even after adjusting for those factors that increased the teenager's risk for pregnancy, such as growing up in poverty, having parents with low levels of education, growing up in a single-parent family, and having low attachment to and performance in school.

A CDC Priority: Reducing Teen Pregnancy And Promoting Health Equity Among Youth

Teen pregnancy prevention is one of CDC's top six priorities, a "Winnable Battle" in public health and of paramount importance to health and quality of life for our youth. Evidence-based teen pregnancy prevention programs typically address specific protective factors on the basis of knowledge, skills, beliefs, or attitudes related to teen pregnancy.

1. Knowledge of sexual issues, human immunodeficiency virus (HIV), other STDs, and pregnancy (including methods of prevention).

2. Perception of HIV risk.

3. Personal values about sex and abstinence.

4. Attitudes toward condoms (pro and con).

5. Perception of peer norms and behavior about sex.

6. Individual ability to refuse sex and to use condoms.

7. Intent to abstain from sex, or limit number of partners.

8. Communication with parents or other adults about sex, condoms, and contraception.

9. Individual ability to avoid HIV/STD risk and risk behaviors.

10. Avoidance of places and situations that might lead to sex.

11. Intent to use a condom.

Non-Hispanic black youth, Hispanic/Latino youth, American Indian/Alaska Native youth, and socioeconomically disadvantaged youth of any race or ethnicity experience the highest rates of teen pregnancy and childbirth. Together, black and Hispanic youth comprise nearly 60% of U.S. teen births in 2008. CDC is focusing on these priority populations because of the need for greater public health efforts to improve the life trajectories of adolescents facing significant health disparities, as well as to have the greatest impact on overall U.S. teen birth rates. Other priority populations for CDC's teen pregnancy prevention efforts include youth in foster care and the juvenile justice systems, and otherwise living in conditions of risk.

Reducing Teen Pregnancy In 2010–2015

As part of the President's Teen Pregnancy Prevention Initiative (TPPI), CDC is partnering with the U.S. Department of Health and Human Services, Office of Public Health and Science (OPHS) to reduce teen pregnancy and address disparities in teen pregnancy and birth rates. The OPHS Office of Adolescent Health (OAH) supports public and private entities to fund medically accurate and age-appropriate evidence-based or innovative program models to reduce teen pregnancy.

TPPI is focused on communities with the highest rates of teen pregnancy, with an emphasis on reaching African American and Hispanic/Latino youth. In order to reduce community-wide teen pregnancy and birth rates, programs will need to use broad-based strategies that reach a majority of youth in the community, as well as more intensive strategies customized to reach youth at highest risk for teen pregnancy.

Program goals are the following:

1. Reduce the rates of teen pregnancies and births in the target area.

2. Increase youth access to evidence-based and evidence-informed programs to prevent teen pregnancy.

3. Increase linkages between teen pregnancy prevention programs and community-based clinical services.

4. Educate stakeholders about relevant evidence-based and evidence-informed strategies to reduce teen pregnancy, and on needs and resources in target communities.

In 2010, CDC issued two competitive funding opportunity announcements to support cooperative agreements with community-based organizations and national organizations for 2010 through 2015:

1. A joint CDC and OPHS funding opportunity for up to $10 million from the TPPI to support community-based organizations to fund demonstration projects to test innovative, sustainable, community-wide multi-component initiatives. This announcement also makes available $2 million in CDC funds to support national organizations that will provide training and technical assistance to the community-based projects.

2. CDC issued a funding announcement providing up to $1,000,000 in funds under Title X of the Public Health Service Act to support an additional community-based project.

These programs will build upon experience from the past. From 2005 through 2010, CDC funded nine state teen pregnancy prevention organizations, four Title X Regional Training Centers, and three national teen pregnancy prevention organizations through the Promoting Science-Based Approaches to Prevent Teen Pregnancy (PSBA) program. Through intensive training and technical assistance, state and local youth-serving organizations built their capacity to provide youth with evidence-based teen pregnancy prevention programming, and to evaluate and sustain these efforts. From 2007 through 2009, in school- and community-based settings, more than 50,000 youth received evidence-based comprehensive sex education curricula and/or youth development programming shown to prevent teen pregnancy or reduce associated behavioral risk factors.

Chapter 5

Questions And Answers About Sexuality Education

Sexuality education is a lifelong process of acquiring information and forming attitudes, beliefs, and values. It encompasses sexual development, sexual and reproductive health, interpersonal relationships, affection, intimacy, body image, and gender roles.

Where do young people learn about sexuality?

Sexuality education begins at home. Parents and caregivers are—and ought to be—the primary sexuality educators of their children. Teachable moments—opportunities to discuss sexuality issues with children—occur on a daily basis.

From the moment of birth, children learn about love, touch, and relationships. Infants and toddlers learn about sexuality when their parents talk to them, dress them, show affection, and teach them the names of the parts of their bodies. As children grow into adolescence, they continue to receive messages about sexual behaviors, attitudes, and values from their families.

Young people also learn about sexuality from other sources such as friends, television, music, books, advertisements, and the internet. And, they frequently learn through planned opportunities in faith communities, community-based agencies, and schools.

What are the goals of school-based sexuality education?

The primary goal of school-based sexuality education is to help young people build a foundation as they mature into sexually healthy adults. School-based sexuality education should

About This Chapter: Information in this chapter is from "Sexuality Education Questions and Answers," published by SIECUS, the Sexuality Information and Education Council of the United States, www.siecus.org. © 2011. Reprinted with permission.

be designed to complement and augment the sexuality education children receive from their families, religious and community groups, and health care professionals. Such programs should respect the diversity of values and beliefs represented in the community.

Sexuality education should assist young people in understanding a positive view of sexuality, provide them with information and skills for taking care of their sexual health, and help them make sound decisions now and in the future.

Comprehensive sexuality education programs have four main goals:

- To provide accurate information about human sexuality

- To provide an opportunity for young people to develop and understand their values, attitudes, and insights about sexuality

- To help young people develop relationships and interpersonal skills, and

- To help young people exercise responsibility regarding sexual relationships, which includes addressing abstinence, pressures to become prematurely involved in sexual intercourse, and the use of contraception and other sexual health measures.

How do school-based sexuality education programs differ?

When discussing the sexuality education young people receive, many people refer to two distinct schools of thought: comprehensive sexuality education and abstinence-only-until-marriage programs. In reality, however, most schools in the United States teach programs that fall somewhere between the two ends of the spectrum and programs are often called by a variety of different names.

The following terms and definitions provide a basic understanding of the types of sexuality education programs that are currently offered in schools and communities. Remember, however, that names can be deceiving. It is important to look past labels and find out what young people in your community really are, or are not, learning in their sexuality education programs.

- **Comprehensive Sexuality Education:** Sexuality education programs that start in kindergarten and continue through 12th grade. These programs include age-appropriate, medically accurate information on a broad set of topics related to sexuality including human development, relationships, decision-making, abstinence, contraception, and disease prevention. They provide students with opportunities for developing skills as well as learning information.

- **Abstinence Based:** Programs that emphasize the benefits of abstinence. These programs also include information about sexual behavior other than intercourse as well as contraception and disease prevention methods. These programs are also referred to as abstinence plus or abstinence centered.

- **Abstinence Only:** Programs that emphasize abstinence from all sexual behaviors. These programs do not include information about contraception or disease prevention methods.

- **Abstinence Only Until Marriage:** Programs that emphasize abstinence from all sexual behaviors outside of marriage. If contraception or disease-prevention methods are discussed, these programs typically emphasize failure rates. In addition, they often present marriage as the only morally correct context for sexual activity.

- **Fear Based:** Abstinence-only and abstinence-only-until-marriage programs that are designed to control young people's sexual behavior by instilling fear, shame, and guilt. These programs rely on negative messages about sexuality, distort information about condoms and sexually transmitted diseases (STDs), and promote biases based on gender, sexual orientation, marriage, family structure, and pregnancy options.

Ideally, what topics are included in comprehensive sexuality education?

In 1991, the Sexuality Information and Education Council of the United States (SIECUS) convened the National Guidelines Task Force, bringing together experts in the fields of adolescent development, sexuality, and education. The task force identified six key concept areas that should be part of any comprehensive sexuality education program: human development, relationships, personal skills, sexual behavior, sexual health, and society and culture.

The Task Force published the *Guidelines for Comprehensive Sexuality Education: K–12*, a framework designed to help educators and communities create new programs and evaluate existing curricula. Now in its third edition, the Guidelines provide age-appropriate messages about 39 topics related to sexuality for school-age young people. (See SIECUS Guidelines www.siecus.org/pubs/guidelines/guidelines.pdf)

What are students learning in today's school-based sexuality education?

The content of sexuality education varies depending on the community and the age of the students in the programs. Unfortunately, there is not enough research done each year to give us an accurate picture of what young people are and are not learning in sexuality education courses.

A recent study of health education programs conducted by the Centers for Disease Control and Prevention's (CDC) Division of Adolescent and School Health, however, provides some insight into what is being taught in America's classroom. The study found that 86 percent of all high schools taught about abstinence as the most effective way to avoid pregnancy and STDs, 82 percent taught about risks associated with multiple partners, 77 percent taught about human development topics (such as reproductive anatomy and puberty), 79 percent taught about dating and relationships, 65 percent taught about condom efficacy, 69 percent taught about marriage and commitment, 48 percent taught about sexual identity and sexual orientation, and 39 percent taught students how to correctly use a condom.

In 2002, other researchers asked students what formal instruction they had received in sexuality education topics and found that one-third of teens had not received any formal instruction about contraception. More than 20 percent of both males and females reported receiving abstinence instruction without receiving instruction on birth control, and only 62 percent of sexually experienced female teens reported receiving instruction about contraception before they first had sex.

Quick Tip

Parents and advocates who want to know exactly what is being taught in their schools should contact school administrators, their school board, or teachers.

What does the research say about comprehensive sexuality education?

Numerous studies and evaluations published in peer-reviewed literature have found that comprehensive education about sexuality—programs that teach teens about both abstinence and contraception/disease prevention—is an effective strategy to help young people delay their initiation of sexual intercourse.

Reviews of published evaluations of sexuality education, human immunodeficiency virus (HIV)-prevention, and adolescent pregnancy-prevention programs have consistently found that they:

- do not encourage teens to start having sexual intercourse

- do not increase the frequency with which teens have intercourse, and

- do not increase the number of sexual partners teens have.

Instead these programs can:

- delay the onset of intercourse
- reduce the number of sexual partners, and
- reduce the frequency of intercourse
- increase condom or contraceptive use.

Who decides what young people learn in sexuality education classes?

Individuals and agencies at the federal, state, and local level—from state lawmakers to school board committees to classroom teachers—are all involved in the decisions that ultimately determine what young people learn in the classroom.

The federal government does not have a direct role in local sexuality education. Instead, it leaves such control to state and local bodies. However, because the federal government does control funding for many educational programs, it can influence programs in local schools and communities.

States are much more directly involved in decisions about sexuality education. States can mandate that sexuality education be taught, require schools to teach about STDs or HIV/ acquired immune deficiency syndrome (AIDS), set statewide guidelines for topics, choose curricula, and approve textbooks.

The majority of decisions about education policy, however, are made at the local level.

On the local level, decisions are made by school boards, administrators, and teachers. Many districts have also created special advisory committees to review the materials used in school health and sexuality education courses. Most often these committees make recommendations to the school board which the board can either accept or reject. Teachers, clergy, public health officials, parents, and students often serve on such advisory committees.

It's A Fact!

Whether or not there is a state course or content mandate in place, local administrators may establish their own mandates. These local mandates may expand upon but cannot violate state mandates. If a state mandates that schools provide information on contraception and STD prevention, a local community cannot choose to implement a solely abstinence-only-until-marriage program that does not contain this information. In contrast, if a state prohibits schools from providing contraception and STD prevention information in favor of an abstinence-only-until-marriage message, schools cannot choose to include that information in their programs.

Birth Control Methods

There is no best method of birth control. Each method has its pros and cons.

All women and men can have control over when, and if, they become parents. Making choices about birth control, or contraception, isn't easy. There are many things to think about. To get started, learn about birth control methods you or your partner can use to prevent pregnancy. You can also talk with your doctor about the choices.

Keep in mind, even the most effective birth control methods can fail. But your chances of getting pregnant are lowest if the method you choose always is used correctly and every time you have sex.

Types Of Birth Control

Continuous Abstinence

This means not having sex (vaginal, anal, or oral) at any time. It is the only sure way to prevent pregnancy and protect against sexually transmitted infections (STIs), including human immunodeficiency virus (HIV).

Barrier Methods

These methods put up a block, or barrier, to keep sperm from reaching the egg.

Contraceptive Sponge: This barrier method is a soft, disk-shaped device with a loop for taking it out. It is made out of polyurethane foam and contains the spermicide nonoxynol-9. Spermicide kills sperm.

About This Chapter: Information in this chapter is from "Birth Control Methods: Frequently Asked Questions," U.S. Department of Health and Human Services, March 2009.

It's A Fact!

Only one kind of contraceptive sponge is sold in the United States. It is called the Today Sponge. Women who are sensitive to the spermicide nonoxynol-9 should not use the sponge.

Diaphragm, Cervical Cap, And Cervical Shield: These barrier methods block the sperm from entering the cervix (the opening to your womb) and reaching the egg. The diaphragm is a shallow latex cup. The cervical cap is a thimble-shaped latex cup. It often is called by its brand name, FemCap. The cervical shield is a silicone cup that has a one-way valve that creates suction and helps it fit against the cervix. It often is called by its brand name, Lea's Shield.

Female Condom: This condom is worn by the woman inside her vagina. It keeps sperm from getting into her body. It is made of thin, flexible, manmade rubber and is packaged with a lubricant. It can be inserted up to eight hours before having sex. Use a new condom each time you have intercourse. And don't use it and a male condom at the same time.

Male Condom: Male condoms are a thin sheath placed over an erect penis to keep sperm from entering a woman's body. Condoms can be made of latex, polyurethane, or natural/lambskin. The natural kind do not protect against STIs. Condoms work best when used with a vaginal spermicide, which kills the sperm. And you need to use a new condom with each sex act.

Condoms are one of the following:

- Lubricated, which can make sexual intercourse more comfortable

- Nonlubricated, which can also be used for oral sex. It is best to add lubrication to nonlubricated condoms if you use them for vaginal or anal sex. You can use a water-based lubricant, such as K-Y jelly. You can buy them at the drug store. Oil-based lubricants like massage oils, baby oil, lotions, or petroleum jelly will weaken the condom, causing it to tear or break.

Hormonal Methods

These methods prevent pregnancy by interfering with ovulation, fertilization, and/or implantation of the fertilized egg.

Oral Contraceptives (Combined Pill): The pill contains the hormones estrogen and progestin. It is taken daily to keep the ovaries from releasing an egg. The pill also causes changes in the lining of the uterus and the cervical mucus to keep the sperm from joining the egg.

Quick Tip

Keep condoms in a cool, dry place. If you keep them in a hot place (like a wallet or glove compartment), the latex breaks down. Then the condom can tear or break.

Oral Contraceptives (Progestin-Only Pill, Mini-Pill): Unlike the pill, the mini-pill only has one hormone—progestin. Taken daily, the mini-pill thickens cervical mucus, which keeps the sperm from joining the egg. Less often, it stops the ovaries from releasing an egg.

The Patch: Also called by its brand name, Ortho Evra, this skin patch is worn on the lower abdomen, buttocks, outer arm, or upper body. It releases the hormones progestin and estrogen into the bloodstream to stop the ovaries from releasing eggs in most women. It also thickens the cervical mucus, which keeps the sperm from joining with the egg. You put on a new patch once a week for three weeks. You don't use a patch the fourth week in order to have a period.

Shot/Injection: The birth control shot often is called by its brand name Depo-Provera. With this method you get injections, or shots, of the hormone progestin in the buttocks or arm every three months. A new type is injected under the skin. The birth control shot stops the ovaries from releasing an egg in most women. It also causes changes in the cervix that keep the sperm from joining with the egg.

Vaginal Ring: This is a thin, flexible ring that releases the hormones progestin and estrogen. It works by stopping the ovaries from releasing eggs. It also thickens the cervical mucus, which keeps the sperm from joining the egg.

It is commonly called NuvaRing, its brand name. You squeeze the ring between your thumb and index finger and insert it into your vagina. You wear the ring for three weeks, take it out for the week that you have your period, and then put in a new ring.

Implantable Devices

Implantable devices are inserted into the body and left in place for a few years.

It's A Fact!

The shot should not be used more than two years in a row because it can cause a temporary loss of bone density.

31

Implantable Rod: This is a matchstick-sized, flexible rod that is put under the skin of the upper arm. It is often called by its brand name, Implanon. The rod releases progestin, which causes changes in the lining of the uterus and the cervical mucus to keep the sperm from joining an egg. Less often, it stops the ovaries from releasing eggs. It is effective for up to three years.

Intrauterine Devices Or IUDs: An IUD is a small device shaped like a T that goes in your uterus. There are two types: copper IUD and hormonal IUD.

Permanent Birth Control Methods

Permanent methods are for people who are sure they never want to have a child or do not want more children.

Sterilization Implant (Essure): Essure is the first nonsurgical method of sterilizing women. A thin tube is used to thread a tiny spring-like device through the vagina and uterus into each fallopian tube. The device works by causing scar tissue to form around the coil. This blocks the fallopian tubes and stops the egg and sperm from joining.

Surgical Sterilization: For women, surgical sterilization closes the fallopian tubes by being cut, tied, or sealed. This stops the eggs from going down to the uterus where they can be fertilized. The surgery can be done a number of ways. Sometimes, a woman having cesarean birth has the procedure done at the same time, so as to avoid having additional surgery later.

For men, having a vasectomy keeps sperm from going to his penis, so his ejaculate never has any sperm in it. Sperm stays in the system after surgery for about three months. During that time, use a backup form of birth control to prevent pregnancy. A simple test can be done to check if all the sperm is gone; it is called a semen analysis.

Emergency Contraception (Morning After Pill)

Emergency birth control is used to keep a woman from getting pregnant when she has had unprotected vaginal intercourse. Unprotected can mean that no method of birth control was used. It can also mean that a birth control method was used but did not work—like a condom breaking. Or, a woman may have forgotten to take her birth control pills, or may have been abused or forced to have sex.

Emergency contraception consists of taking two doses of hormonal pills 12 hours apart. They work by stopping the ovaries from releasing an egg or keeping the sperm from joining with the egg. For the best chances for it to work, start the pills as soon as possible after unprotected sex. It should be started within 72 hours after having unprotected sex. It should not be used as a regular method of birth control.

Birth Control And Sexually Transmitted Infections (STIs)

The male latex condom is the only birth control method proven to help protect you from STIs, including HIV. Research is being done to find out how effective the female condom is at preventing STIs and HIV.

Effectiveness

All birth control methods work best if used correctly and every time you have sex. Be sure you know the right way to use them. Sometimes doctors don't explain how to use a method because they assume you already know. Talk with your doctor if you have questions. Doctors are used to talking about birth control. So don't feel embarrassed about talking to him or her.

Some birth control methods can take time and practice to learn. For example, some people don't know you can put on a male condom inside out. Also, not everyone knows you need to leave a little space at the tip of the condom for the sperm and fluid when a man ejaculates, or has an orgasm.

Getting Birth Control

Where you get birth control depends on what method you choose. You can buy the following forms over the counter: male condoms, female condoms, sponges, spermicides, and emergency contraception pills (girls younger than 17 need a prescription).

You need a prescription for the following forms: oral contraceptives (the pill, the mini-pill); skin patch; vaginal ring; diaphragm (your doctor needs to fit one to your shape); cervical cap; cervical shield; shot/injection (you get the shot at your doctor's office); IUD (inserted by a doctor); implantable rod (inserted by a doctor).

Spermicides

You can buy spermicides over the counter. They work by killing sperm. They come in many forms: foam, gel, cream, film, suppository, and tablet.

Spermicides are put in the vagina no more than one hour before having sex. If you use a film, suppository, or tablet, wait at least 15 minutes before having sex so the spermicide can dissolve. Do not douche or rinse out your vagina for at least six to eight hours after having sex. You will need to use more spermicide each time you have sex.

Spermicides work best if used along with a barrier method, such as a condom, diaphragm, or cervical cap. Some spermicides are made just for use with the diaphragm and cervical cap. Check the package to make sure you are buying what you need.

Withdrawal

Withdrawal is when a man takes his penis out of a woman's vagina (or pulls out) before he ejaculates, or has an orgasm. This stops the sperm from going to the egg. Pulling out can be hard for a man to do. It takes a lot of self-control, and it is not a very effective method of birth control.

Even if you use withdrawal, sperm can be released before the man pulls out. When a man's penis first becomes erect, preejaculate fluid may be on the tip of the penis. This fluid has sperm in it. So you could still get pregnant.

It's A Fact!
Withdrawal does not protect you from STIs or HIV.

Chapter 7

Teen Pregnancy And The Media

This chapter presents new polling data on teens' opinions about media and teen pregnancy in general, as well as their views about MTV's popular *16 and Pregnant* program in particular. Some have criticized this show and others like it for glamorizing teen pregnancy. These results suggest that teens have a different view. The overwhelming majority of teens report that shows dealing with teen pregnancy make them think about their own risks of getting pregnant or causing a pregnancy and that *16 and Pregnant* helps young people better understand the challenges of pregnancy and parenting.

Methodology

The following results are drawn from a public opinion poll of 1,008 young people ages 12–19. Interviews were conducted by phone and took place between August 12 and September 12, 2010. The survey is weighted to provide a nationally representative estimate of young people 12–19. The sample for this survey was drawn using two different methods: random digit dialing of households with telephones and from a database of households with young people ages 12–19. The margin of error is +/-3.09 at the 95% confidence level. The survey was commissioned and designed by The National Campaign to Prevent Teen and Unplanned Pregnancy and was conducted by Social Science Research Solutions (www.ssrs.com), a division of International Communications Research.

About This Chapter: Information in this chapter is from "Does the Media Glamorize Teen Pregnancy?" © 2010 The National Campaign to Prevent Teen Pregnancy. Reprinted with permission. For additional information, visit www.thenationalcampaign.org.

Headlines

- Most teens (79% of girls and 67% of boys) say that when a TV show or character they like deals with teen pregnancy, it makes them think more about their own risk of getting pregnant or causing a pregnancy and how to avoid it.

- Among those teens who have watched MTV's *16 and Pregnant*, 82% think the show helps teens better understand the challenges of teen pregnancy and parenthood.

- Just 15% who've seen the show believe it glamorizes teen pregnancy.

- Three-quarters of teens (76%) say that what they see in the media about sex, love, and relationships can be a good way to start conversations with adults. About half (48%) say they sometimes or often have conversations about these topics with their parents because of something they've seen in the media.

Detailed Findings

Please Note: All the responses are for young people ages 12–19. Due to rounding, the numbers in these charts might not add to the net number presented.

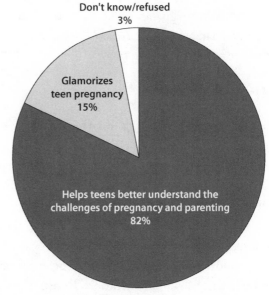

Teens (aged 12-19)

Figure 7.1. Question: Teen pregnancy has been the focus of many entertainment programs recently. Thinking specifically about MTV's 16 and Pregnant, do you think the show helps teens better understand the challenges of pregnancy and parenthood or does it glamorize teen pregnancy?

Note: 39% of teens surveyed had not seen the show. Boys were much more likely than girls to report that they had not seen the show (49% versus 29%). However, among those teens who have seen the show, the reactions to the show were the same for both boys and girls.

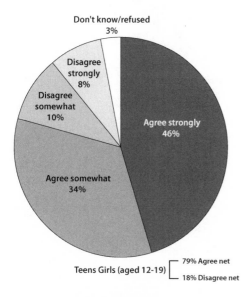

Don't know/refused
3%

Disagree strongly
8%

Disagree somewhat
10%

Agree strongly
46%

Agree somewhat
34%

Teens Girls (aged 12-19) — 79% Agree net / 18% Disagree net

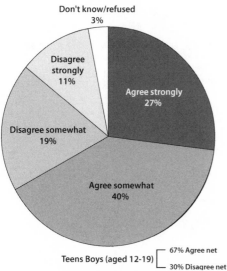

Don't know/refused
3%

Disagree strongly
11%

Disagree somewhat
19%

Agree strongly
27%

Agree somewhat
40%

Teens Boys (aged 12-19) — 67% Agree net / 30% Disagree net

Figure 7.2. (left two charts) *Question:* How much do you agree or disagree with the following statement: When a TV show or character I like deals with teen pregnancy, it makes me think more about my own risk of getting pregnant/causing a pregnancy and how to avoid it.

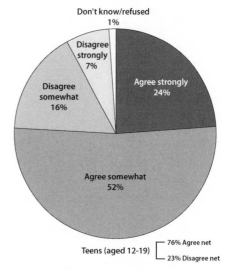

Don't know/refused
1%

Disagree strongly
7%

Disagree somewhat
16%

Agree strongly
24%

Agree somewhat
52%

Teens (aged 12-19) — 76% Agree net / 23% Disagree net

Figure 7.3. (top) *Question:* Stories and events in TV shows and other media about sex, love, and relationships can be a good way to start conversations with adults about these topics. Do you agree or disagree?

Figure 7.4. (bottom) *Question:* How often would you say you and your parents have talked about sex, love, and relationships because of something you saw in popular media (like television shows)?

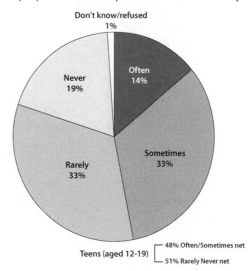

Don't know/refused
1%

Never
19%

Often
14%

Rarely
33%

Sometimes
33%

Teens (aged 12-19) — 48% Often/Sometimes net / 51% Rarely Never net

37

Part Two
If You Think You're Pregnant

Chapter 8

Finding Out If You're Pregnant

Pregnancy symptoms differ from woman to woman and pregnancy to pregnancy; however, one of the most significant pregnancy symptoms is a delayed or missed menstrual cycle.

Understanding the signs and symptoms of pregnancy is important because each symptom may be related to something other than pregnancy. Some women experience signs or symptoms of pregnancy within a week of conception. For other women, pregnancy symptoms may develop over a few weeks or may not be present at all.

Below is a listing of some of the most common pregnancy signs and symptoms. If you have been sexually active and are experiencing any of the following symptoms, it is important to take a pregnancy test.

Implantation Bleeding

Implantation bleeding can be one of the earliest pregnancy symptoms. About 6–12 days after conception, the embryo implants itself into the uterine wall. Some women will experience spotting as well as some cramping.

Other Explanations: Actual menstruation, altered menstruation, changes in birth control pill, infection, or abrasion from intercourse.

Delay/Difference In Menstruation

A delayed or missed period is the most common pregnancy symptom leading a woman to test for pregnancy. When you become pregnant, your next period should be missed. Many

About This Chapter: Information in this chapter is from "Pregnancy Symptoms—Early Signs of Pregnancy," © 2011 American Pregnancy Association (www.americanpregnancy.org). Reprinted with permission.

women can bleed while they are pregnant, but typically the bleeding will be shorter or lighter than a normal period.

Other Explanations: Excessive weight gain/loss, fatigue, hormonal problems, tension, stress, ceasing to take the birth control pill, illness, or breastfeeding.

Swollen/Tender Breasts

Swollen or tender breasts is a pregnancy symptom which may begin as early as one to two weeks after conception. Women may notice changes in their breasts; they may be tender to the touch, sore, or swollen.

Other Explanations: Hormonal imbalance, birth control pills, impending menstruation (premenstrual syndrome, or PMS) can also cause your breasts to be swollen or tender.

Fatigue/Tiredness

Feeling fatigued or more tired is a pregnancy symptom which can also start as early as the first week after conception.

Other Explanations: Stress, exhaustion, depression, common cold or flu, or other illnesses can also leave you feeling tired or fatigued.

Nausea/Morning Sickness

This well known pregnancy symptom will often show up between two to eight weeks after conception. Some women are fortunate to not deal with morning sickness at all, while others will feel nauseous throughout most of their pregnancy.

Other Explanations: Food poisoning, stress, change in hormonal birth control method, or other stomach disorders can also cause you to feel queasy.

Backaches

Lower backaches may be a symptom that occurs early in pregnancy; however, it is common to experience a dull backache throughout pregnancy.

Other Explanations: Impending menstruation, stress, other back problems, and physical or mental strains.

Headaches

The sudden rise of hormones in your body can cause you to have headaches early in pregnancy.

Other Explanations: Dehydration, caffeine withdrawal, impending menstruation, eye strain, or other ailments can be the source of frequent or chronic headaches.

Frequent Urination

Around six to eight weeks after conception, you may find yourself making a few extra trips to the bathroom.

Other Explanations: Urinary tract infection, diabetes, increasing liquid intake, or taking excessive diuretics.

Home Pregnancy Tests (HPTs)

HPTs are inexpensive, private, and easy to use. Most drugstores sell HPTs over the counter. The cost depends on the brand and how many tests come in the box. They work by detecting human chorionic gonadotropin (hCG) in your urine. HPTs are highly accurate. But their accuracy depends on many things. These include the following:

- **When You Use Them:** The amount of hCG in your urine increases with time. So, the earlier after a missed period you take the test the harder it is to spot the hCG. Some HPTs claim that they can tell if you are pregnant one day after a missed period or even earlier. But a recent study shows that most HPTs don't give accurate results this early in pregnancy. Positive results are more likely to be true than negative results. Waiting one week after a missed period will usually give a more accurate result.

- **How You Use Them:** Be sure to check the expiration date and follow the directions. Many involve holding a test stick in the urine stream. For some, you collect urine in a cup and then dip the test stick into it. Then, depending on the brand, you will wait a few minutes to get the results. Research suggests waiting 10 minutes will give the most accurate result. Also, testing your urine first thing in the morning may boost the accuracy.

- **Who Uses Them:** The amount of hCG in the urine is different for every pregnant woman. So, some women will have accurate results on the day of the missed period while others will need to wait longer. Also, some medicines affect HPTs. Discuss the medicines you use with your doctor before trying to become pregnant.

- **The Brand Of Test:** Some HPT tests are better than others at spotting hCG early on.

The most important part of using any HPT is to follow the directions exactly as written. Most tests also have toll-free phone numbers to call in case of questions about use or results.

If a HPT says you are pregnant, you should call your doctor right away. Your doctor can use a more sensitive test along with a pelvic exam to tell for sure if you're pregnant. Seeing your doctor early on in your pregnancy can help you and your baby stay healthy.

Source: From "Knowing If You Are Pregnant," a publication of the Office on Women's Health, U.S. Department of Health and Human Services, September 2010.

Darkening Of Areolas

If you are pregnant, the skin around your nipples may get darker.

Other Explanations: Hormonal imbalance unrelated to pregnancy or may be a leftover effect from a previous pregnancy.

Food Cravings Or Food Aversions

While you may not have a strong desire to eat pickles and ice cream, many women will feel cravings for certain foods when they are pregnant. This can last throughout your entire pregnancy. Some women develop aversions to certain types of food early in pregnancy and this too can last for the next nine months.

Other Explanations: Poor diet, lack of a certain nutrient, stress, depression, illness, or impending menstruation.

Chapter 9

Telling Parents You're Pregnant

It's been three days since she got the results, but Tina still can't believe her pregnancy test came out positive. She can't get it off her mind. It feels like her whole life has changed. She knows she has to tell her parents. But she's not sure she's prepared for how they might react.

Confused? You're Not Alone

If you've just learned you're pregnant, you're not alone.

You might feel confused, scared, or shocked by the news. You might think, "This can't really be happening." You promise yourself you'll be so much more careful in the future. And you know you'll probably have to tell your parents.

Preparing To Talk To Parents

No matter how close you are to your parents, you're going to wonder how they'll react. It's one thing if your parents realize you're having sex and they're OK with that. But it's another thing if they've forbidden you to date or if having premarital sex is completely against their values and beliefs.

Most parents fall somewhere in the middle. For example, some parents have pretty liberal values but they're still shocked to learn their teen had sex. Even parents who know their teens are having sex can still be disappointed or worried about their future.

About This Chapter: Information in this chapter is from "Telling Parents You're Pregnant," May 2009, reprinted with permission from www.kidshealth.org. Copyright © 2009 The Nemours Foundation. This information was provided by KidsHealth, one of the largest resources online for medically reviewed health information written for parents, kids, and teens. For more articles like this one, visit www.KidsHealth.org, or www.TeensHealth.org.

Your parents' personalities also play a part in how they'll react. Some parents are easy to talk to or calmer in a crisis. Some are more emotional, more easily stressed out, more likely to get upset or angry, to yell or cry, or express themselves loudly.

Most parents want to be supportive of a daughter who is pregnant (or a son who got a girl pregnant), even if they are angry or upset at first. But a few may react violently to the news and let anger get out of control. If you think your parents might fall into this category—for example, if they have a history of physical violence—read the section on Protecting Yourself at the end of this chapter.

Some parents don't show how they feel at first. They may take time to absorb the news. Others react quickly and there's no mistaking how they feel. Some will listen and be sensitive to your feelings. Some parents will spring into action, taking charge and telling you what to do.

Think about how your parents have reacted to other situations. Try to imagine how they might respond—but remember it's impossible to really know for sure. Still, thinking about what to expect can help you feel prepared for the conversation you plan to have.

The Conversation

First, find the words. You might say, "I have something difficult to tell you. I found out that I'm pregnant." Then wait. Allow your parents to absorb what you said.

Be prepared to deal with the reaction. What happens next? Will your parents be angry, stressed, or emotional? Will they lecture you? Use harsh words? Ask a ton of questions?

It's good to think ahead about what you might do and how you may feel. For instance, if a parent yells, you'll want to be prepared so you can keep the conversation productive and resist any urge to yell back.

Of course, not every parent yells. Many don't. Even if parents have a strong reaction at first, most want to help their children. Lots of teens are surprised at how supportive their parents turn out to be.

It can help to tell your parents that you understand their feelings and point of view. Saying things like, "I know you're really mad," "I know this isn't what you wanted for me," or, "I know this isn't what you expected" can help your parents be more understanding. The key is to be honest and speak from the heart. If you say what you think parents want to hear or make statements just to calm them, it might sound fake.

Give your parents time to speak without jumping in. Listen to what they say. Let them vent if they have to.

Tell them how you feel. Part of your conversation might involve telling parents how you feel. For example, if you know you've disappointed them and you feel sorry about it, say that. Let them know if you feel disappointed in yourself, too.

You might say, "Mom and Dad, I know I've disappointed you. I know you're upset. I'm really sorry for putting you through this. I'm disappointed in myself, too."

Share your fears and worries, such as, "I'm scared about how I'm going to handle this, what my friends will think, and what it means about school." Or, "I can't believe this is happening to me and I'm not sure what to do."

Putting your feelings into words takes plenty of maturity and it's not easy to do. Don't worry if the words don't come out perfectly or if you cry or get emotional as you're saying them. It can help to think about your feelings ahead of time. If you can't imagine expressing your feelings out loud, consider writing them down in a letter.

If you need to, get help breaking the news. A visit to your doctor's office or a health clinic is a must—not just for your health, but to get more information and discuss the realities of your situation. You'll want to understand your choices and explore your feelings with an experienced professional. During your visit, the doctor, nurse, or health counselor also can help you think through how to tell your parents. If you want, they could even be there as you talk to your parents.

Talking About Your Decisions

Now that you've told your parents, you'll have some important decisions to make. Talking decisions over with others can help. Sometimes parents—including your boyfriend's parents—can offer a new angle or ideas.

It's A Fact!

Lots of things will influence how a parent reacts to news of your pregnancy, such as:

- how surprised or shocked your parents might be to learn you've been having sex
- your parents' values about dating, sex, and pregnancy
- your parents' expectations or rules for you
- your parents' feelings about your partner and your relationship
- your age or maturity level

Whatever you decide, it needs to be what you want, not what someone else wants you to do. That's especially true if you think most of the child-raising will fall to you. It's a big job.

Becoming a teen parent affects your education, job, and financial future—and often your boyfriend's too. Over half of teen pregnancies end with the birth of the baby. Some teens decide to keep the baby. Others let someone adopt the child. Some teen pregnancies end in miscarriage, and about one third end in abortion.

Talking about your options isn't easy, especially if none of them is what you had in mind. Some families need the help of a counselor to talk about this difficult and complicated situation in a way that lets everyone be respected and heard.

It's More Than Just Breaking The News

Talking to a parent about your pregnancy takes more than just one conversation. In the coming months, you'll probably have many different feelings all at once. Sometimes, you might feel shock and disbelief. Other times, you may be scared or worried. You may feel sad, guilty, or angry at yourself. At times, you might also feel excited and happy.

Some days you might be ready for what's ahead. Other days, you may feel totally unprepared and confused. You'll have many emotions to sort through and it will take time. It helps if you can talk to a parent about all these thoughts and feelings.

Protecting Yourself

To some parents, the news that you're having a baby will feel like a terrible crisis. Depending on their beliefs, cultural values, or personalities, parents might feel shame, guilt, or embarrassment. They might feel angry and assign blame. Sometimes parents scream, yell, and use putdowns. In some cases, anger can get out of control.

You know your parent and you know your situation. If you need to tell your parents you're pregnant but think they might react in a way that could hurt you, have someone else with you when you tell them. If you're concerned about your safety, get advice. A teen health clinic, such as Planned Parenthood, or a teen pregnancy hotline can guide you and steer you toward resources to support you.

Of course, most parents won't react with extreme anger. The thing to remember is every parent is different and you know yours best.

When Parents Have Your Back

Talking to parents whenever you can is a good way to sort through the many feelings and issues that arise. In the best of situations, parents can help you make important decisions and support your choices. They can be a source of guidance and encouragement.

Sometimes a difficult situation brings people closer and strengthens their bonds. Sometimes, however unexpectedly, a difficult situation can help a family discover unconditional love, support, kindness, forgiveness, acceptance, teamwork, and optimism.

Chapter 10

Thinking About Abortion

Millions of women face unplanned pregnancies every year. If you are deciding what to do about an unplanned pregnancy, you have a lot to think about. You have three options—abortion, adoption, and parenting.

Whether you're thinking about having an abortion, you're helping a woman decide if abortion is right for her, or you're just curious about abortion, you may have many questions. Here are some of the most common questions we hear women ask when considering abortion. We hope you find the answers helpful.

How can I know if abortion is the right option for me?

We all have many important decisions to make in life. What to do about an unplanned pregnancy is an important and common decision faced by women. In fact, about half of all women in the U.S. have an unplanned pregnancy at some point in their lives. About four out of 10 women with unplanned pregnancies decide to have abortions. Overall, more than one out of three of all U.S. women will have an abortion by the time they are 45 years old.

Women have abortions because they care about themselves and their families or their future families. The most common reasons a woman decides to have an abortion are

- She is not ready to become a parent.

- She cannot afford a baby.

- She feels that having a baby now would make it too difficult to work, go to school, or care for her children.

- She doesn't want to be a single parent.

- She doesn't want anyone to know she has had sex or is pregnant.

- She feels too young or too immature to have a child.

- She has all the children she wants.

- She or the fetus has a health problem.

- She is a survivor of rape or incest.

Every woman's situation is different, and only you can decide what is best in your case. If you're trying to decide if abortion is the right option for you, you may find it helpful to list the advantages and disadvantages of having an abortion. Think about what advantages or disadvantages are most important to you. Consider how you feel and what you think about abortion, what you want for your life and for your family or future family.

Some Things To Ask Yourself If You Are Thinking About Abortion

- Am I ready to become a parent?
- Can I afford to have a child?
- Can I afford to have an abortion?
- Would I prefer to have a child at another time?
- What would it mean for my future and my family's future if I had a child now?
- Would I consider putting the child up for adoption?
- Do I have strong religious beliefs about abortion?
- How do I feel about other women who have abortions?
- How important is it to me what other people will think about my decision?
- Can I handle the experience of having an abortion?
- Is anyone pressuring me to have an abortion? Am I being pressured not to have an abortion?
- Would I be willing to tell a parent or go before a judge if my state requires it?

Think about what your answers mean to you. You may want to discuss your answers with your partner, someone in your family, a friend, a trusted religious adviser, or a counselor.

Who can help me decide?

Women can feel alone or isolated when they are considering abortion. You may feel that it's hard to talk to the people you normally reach out to for support. Some people can be very judgmental. When you're around judgmental people, you may feel bad about yourself or your decisions. Seek out people you know will support you and who will understand that you're trying to do what's best for yourself and your family or future family.

Most women look to their husbands, partners, families, health care providers, clergy, or someone else they trust for support as they make their decision about an unplanned pregnancy. And many women go to the clinic with their partners. But you don't have to tell anybody. If you're 18 or older, it is entirely up to you who you tell.

If You Are A Teen

Teens are encouraged to involve parents in their decision to have an abortion, and most do have a parent involved. But telling a parent is only required in states with mandatory parental involvement laws. Such laws force a woman under 18 to tell a parent or get parental permission before having an abortion. In most of these states, if she can't talk with her parents—or doesn't want to—she can appear before a judge. The judge will consider whether she's mature enough to decide on her own. If not, the judge will decide whether an abortion is in her best interests.

In any case, if there are complications during the abortion, parents of a minor may be notified.

Specially trained educators at women's health clinics—like your Planned Parenthood health center—can talk with you in private. Or you may bring someone with you if you wish. When choosing a clinic, beware of so-called "crisis pregnancy centers" that are run by people who are against abortion.

How soon do I have to decide?

Abortion is safe, and serious complications are rare—but the risk to your health increases the longer a pregnancy continues. Abortions performed later in pregnancy may be more complicated but are still safer than labor and childbirth. So, even though it's important to take the time you need to make the decision that's best for you, it is important that you understand there may be greater health risks later in pregnancy. So, you may not want to wait too long.

How is abortion done?

If you decide to end a pregnancy, your health care provider may talk with you about different abortion methods. You may be offered the option to have an in-clinic abortion, or you may be offered the abortion pill.

Are there any long-term risks of abortion?

There are many myths about the risks of abortion. Here are the facts. Abortion does not cause breast cancer. Safe, uncomplicated abortion does not cause problems for future pregnancies such as birth defects, premature birth or low birth weight babies, ectopic pregnancy, miscarriage, or infant death.

If I have an abortion, how will I feel afterward?

A range of emotions is normal after an abortion. There is not one "correct" way to feel. Some women feel anger, regret, guilt, or sadness for a little while. For some women, these feelings may be quite strong.

For some women, having an abortion can be a significant life event, like ending a relationship, starting or losing a job, or becoming a parent. It can be very stressful and difficult. Other women have an easier time after abortion.

Serious, long-term emotional problems after abortion are about as uncommon as they are after giving birth. They are more likely to happen for certain reasons—for instance, if a woman has a history of emotional problems before the abortion, if she doesn't have supportive people in her life, or if she has to terminate a wanted pregnancy because her health or the health of her fetus is in danger.

Ultimately, most women feel relief after an abortion. Women tend to feel better after abortion if they can talk with supportive people in their lives.

Chapter 11

Thinking About Adoption

The decision to place a child for adoption is never easy. Like the decision to parent a child, it takes courage and much love. Once an adoption is finalized, it is permanent, and it will change your relationship with your child forever. The adoptive parents will raise your child and have full legal rights as the child's parents.

You may want to think about the following questions as you make your decision.

Have I explored all my options?

Pregnancy can affect your feelings and emotions. Are you thinking about adoption only because you have money problems, or because your living situation is difficult? If so, there might be other answers. Have you called Social Services to see what they can do? Have you asked friends and family if they can help? Social workers may be able to help you find a way to parent your baby if that is your decision. For instance, they may be able to help with finding a place to live or job training.

Have I involved the baby's father in thinking about adoption?

You need to know what the laws in your state say about the father's rights, responsibilities, and role in adoption. Most states require that the father—or the man you think is the father—be told about the baby before the adoption. This is true even if you aren't married to the father. If you are married and your husband is not the baby's father, your husband may still have legal rights, responsibilities, and a role in the adoption.

About This Chapter: Information in this chapter is from "Are You Pregnant and Thinking About Adoption?" a publication of the Child Welfare Information Gateway, March 2007. Available online at www.childwelfare.gov/pubs/f_pregna/index.cfm.

> **Quick Tip**
>
> For more information on laws in your state about consent, read Child Welfare Information Gateway's Consent to Adoption at www.childwelfare.gov/systemwide/laws_policies/statutes/consent.cfm.

Your baby's father (or your husband) may have to sign legal papers agreeing to the adoption—giving legal consent—before you can place your child. There are also laws requiring the father to pay child support if you decide to parent your baby.

In some states, if the parents are not married, the father has a certain amount of time to put his name on the state's putative father registry to claim that he is the baby's father. In other states, the father may be required to take other legal action to claim his rights as a father. If he doesn't do this within a certain amount of time, he may not receive notice of the mother's decision to place the child for adoption. If you don't know the father's name or where he is, some states require that a notice be published before the adoption can be completed. The notice is published in a newspaper in a place where the father is likely to see it. A licensed adoption agency or qualified adoption lawyer can explain to you what is required in your state.

If you're thinking about adoption, your agency or lawyer should be able to explain your state's laws about the father's role. In a few cases, agencies or lawyers have pushed through adoptions without telling the father and getting his consent. In some of these cases, the court has legally overturned the adoption and awarded custody of the baby to the father. Any agency or lawyer working with you must obey the law and obtain the father's consent if needed. If your agency or lawyer is not willing to do this, you may want to go somewhere else.

If you have a good relationship with your baby's father, he may be a source of support for you. You may be able to help each other in making this decision. The father of your baby may be asking some of the same questions about adoption that you are asking.

> **Quick Tip**
>
> For more information about father's rights, read Child Welfare Information Gateway's The Rights of Presumed (Putative) Fathers at www.childwelfare.gov/systemwide/laws_policies/statutes/putative.cfm.

Have I involved my own family and the father's family in the decision?

Your family may be a source of support as you consider what to do, even if the pregnancy has put a strain on your relationship. Besides emotional support, your family may be able to provide money, housing, and other kinds of help. The father's family may be able to help, also.

In a few states, if you are under 16 or 18 years of age (it depends on the state), your own parent or parents may also have to give permission for you to place your baby for adoption. Laws vary, and you need to find out the consent laws in your state.

If you decide to go ahead with adoption, there may even be someone in your family or the father's family who would like to adopt your baby.

How might I feel in 20 years if I place my child for adoption or if I parent my child myself?

While it's impossible to know for sure how you will feel many years from now, you may want to consider the long-term effects of any decision you make. For instance, you may want to think about your future both with and without this child. What were your plans before you became pregnant? How would raising a child or placing a child for adoption change those plans? How might you feel if you go on to have other children and a family of your own?

Why am I placing my child for adoption?

If your answer is because it is what you, or you and the father, think is best for yourselves and the baby, then it may be a good decision. It's important to gather all the information you can and to hear the thoughts of your family and friends. In the end, however, you must make a decision you can live with. Don't allow others to pressure you toward one outcome.

Why do some expectant parents choose to place their baby for adoption?

Everyone's situation is different, but many women (and their partners) choose to place their baby because they feel that the baby will have a better life in an adoptive home with parents who may be better prepared to care for a child. These mothers feel that they are putting their baby's best interests ahead of their own by placing their baby with parents who are ready to welcome a child and to love and provide for that child for at least 18 years.

Why do some expectant parents choose to raise their baby rather than place the baby for adoption?

Pregnant women (and their partners) who consider adoption but decide to raise their child themselves may do so because they feel that they have the time, resources, and support from family and friends necessary to raise a child for at least 18 years. They may feel that their biological connection with their child is more important than the advantages that the child might receive from an adoptive home.

When do I have to make the decision?

You don't have to make the final decision about adoption until after your baby is born. You may prepare for adoption, and adoptive parents may be waiting for your child. However, the final and legal decision is made by you, or you and the father, after the child's birth.

Think of it as making the adoption decision twice—once while you are pregnant and then again after the baby is born. It's hard to know what you'll feel like after the birth. This is why most state laws require that the final decision to place a child for adoption be made after the baby is born. As of December 2006, only Alabama and Hawaii allow a birth mother to agree to adoption before the birth of her child. Even in these states, the mother can change her mind after the birth. Some counselors suggest that you wait until you have left the hospital before signing papers that make the adoption final.

Chapter 12

Thinking About Parenting

Millions of women face unplanned pregnancies every year. If you are deciding what to do about an unplanned pregnancy, you have a lot to think about. You have three options—abortion, adoption, and parenting.

Whether you're thinking about parenting, you're helping a woman decide if parenting is right for her, or you're just curious about parenting, you may have many questions. Here are some of the most common questions we hear women ask when considering becoming a parent. We hope you find the answers helpful.

How can I know if parenting is the right option for me?

We all have many important decisions to make in life. What to do about an unplanned pregnancy is an important and common decision faced by women. In fact, about half of all women in the U.S. have an unplanned pregnancy at some point in their lives. About six out of 10 women with unplanned pregnancies decide to continue their pregnancies.

Every woman's situation is different, and only you can decide what is best in your case. If you're trying to decide if parenting is the right option for you, you may find it helpful to list the advantages and disadvantages of having a child. Think about what advantages or disadvantages are most important to you. Consider your feelings and values about raising a child, and what you want for your life and for your family or future family.

About This Chapter: Information in this chapter is reprinted with permission from Planned Parenthood® Federation of America, Inc. © 2011 PPFA. All rights reserved.

What are some of the advantages and disadvantages of parenting?

Though parenting is hard work, it brings many rewards. Being a parent can be exciting and deeply rewarding. It can help you grow, understand yourself better, and enhance your life. Parents can feel delight at their child's accomplishments and the love and bond they share. Many people say that parenting brings great happiness and a deeper understanding of themselves.

But parents often give up a lot for their children. Meeting a child's needs can be very challenging. Parents deal with less sleep and less time to do the things they need and want to do. Having a baby is expensive, and many people find it hard to support their children. Having children can also put a parent's school plans or career on hold.

Many people find that having a child can test even the strongest relationship. And if you are single parenting, you may find it more difficult to find and keep a relationship.

If you already have children, you know firsthand both the joys and challenges parenting can bring. A child will change your life, whether it is your first child or not. If you don't have any children, talking with other parents about their daily lives with their children may help give you an idea about what you could expect.

Some Things To Ask Yourself If You Are Thinking About Raising A Child

- Am I ready to help a child feel wanted and loved?
- Am I ready to cope with a tighter budget, less time for myself, and more stress?
- Do I have the support of family and friends?
- Am I ready to accept responsibility for all my child's needs?
- Would I prefer to have a child at another time?
- Is anyone pressuring me to continue or end the pregnancy?
- How do I feel about other women who have children from unplanned pregnancies?
- Can I afford to have a child?
- What would it mean for my future and my family's future if I had a child now?
- How important is it to me what other people will think about my decision?
- Can I handle the experience of pregnancy and raising a child?

If you are already a parent, ask yourself how bringing another child into your family will affect your other children.

Think about what your answers mean to you. You may want to discuss your answers with your partner, someone in your family, a friend, a trusted religious adviser, or a counselor.

Who can help me decide?

Most women look to their husbands, partners, families, health care providers, clergy, or someone else they trust for support as they make their decision about an unplanned pregnancy. Even though the decision about what to do about your pregnancy is up to you, most women find they'd also like to talk with trusted people in their lives to help them make up their minds.

If you need help deciding, specially trained educators at women's health clinics—like your Planned Parenthood health center—can talk it through with you. They can talk with you in private or you may bring someone with you if you wish. When looking for someone to talk with about your options, beware of so-called "crisis pregnancy centers." They are run by people who are against abortion, and who will not give you information about all of your options.

How soon do I have to decide?

Whether you choose adoption or to become a parent, if there is a chance that you will continue the pregnancy, you should begin prenatal care as soon as possible. You should have a medical exam early in your pregnancy—and regularly throughout your pregnancy—to make sure that you are healthy and the pregnancy is normal.

Even though most women have safe and healthy pregnancies, there are certain risks of pregnancy for a woman. They range from discomforts, such as nausea, fatigue, and aches and pains, to more serious risks, such as blood clots, high blood pressure, and diabetes. In extremely rare cases, complications can be fatal. That's why early and regular prenatal care is very important.

It may be important to take your time and think carefully about your decision. But you may not want to wait too long. If you are considering abortion, you should know that abortion is very safe, but the risks increase the longer a pregnancy goes on.

Can I meet a child's needs?

Children have many needs. Your child will depend on you—for food, shelter, safety, affection, and guidance.

Parenting requires lots of love, energy, and patience. It is often complicated and frustrating. Your child's needs will constantly change and so will your ability to meet those needs. There will be times when you may feel that you are not doing a good job at parenting. To feel good about being a parent, it must be what you want to do—for a long time.

If you are thinking about becoming a parent, you may wonder if you are prepared. Do you have what you might need to take care of a child?

- **Time:** Children can put your school plans or career on hold.

- **Energy And Care:** Children need parents who are loving, patient, and flexible.

- **Planning:** Having children takes daily planning, as well as long-term planning for the next stages of the child's life.

- **Material Things And Money:** Children need clothes, diapers, food, and health care, and they often need day care.

What support will I need if I have a child?

Parenting is hard work—whether you are single and parenting or parenting with a partner, and whether it is your first child or another child in the family. A child requires nonstop care, and having a partner or other family member to share the work of parenting can make the job much easier.

New parents, whether they are single or in a couple, need support from lots of places. Worries about money and time are common for parents, and every family needs support now and then. Sometimes that might be grocery shopping, hand-me-down clothes, babysitting time, or just someone to talk with.

Single Parenting: Many people find themselves single parenting, or choose to become single parents. Single parenting can be very challenging, but it's certainly not impossible.

If you're thinking of single parenting, talk with family and friends about the help you will need. Find out how much time, energy, and money the people in your life are willing to give to you and your baby. If you will need money, be realistic about how much your friends and family can give. Some people will be able to help a lot, while others will be only able to help a little. If you need government support, keep in mind that it will only cover part of what you will need.

But being a single parent has its advantages, too. Because you will not have to make compromises with a partner, you can raise the child as you wish—with your values, principles, and beliefs.

Parenting With A Partner: A partnership can provide parents with much-needed support. Many couples find great satisfaction in sharing the responsibility of raising a child. They find their love and commitment to each other is made deeper by their shared love for their child.

However, parenting can also put stress on relationships. Parents may disagree about what is best for a child. If you have a baby, your relationship with your partner will change. Joint parenting takes good communication and a solid commitment in hard times.

When Extra Support Is Needed

Women often have a wide range of emotions after giving birth. The joy of a new baby can be mixed with feelings of sadness and anxiety, and feelings of being overwhelmed. Childbirth causes sudden shifts in hormones that can cause these feelings. You may need some extra support if you suffer from the "baby blues" during your baby's first few days or weeks.

Long-term depression is more common if a woman has a history of emotional problems or if she does not have supportive people in her life. Women should seek help from a health care provider or counselor if depression lasts more than two weeks or keeps them from doing what they need to do each day.

Overall, having lots of support from other people will be a big help to you if you decide to become a parent. Thinking about how much support you can expect from other people can be very important as you decide what to do about an unplanned pregnancy.

Part Three
Staying Healthy During Your Pregnancy

Chapter 13

Having A Healthy Pregnancy

If you've decided to have a baby, the most important thing you can do is to take good care of yourself so that you and your baby will be healthy. Girls who get the proper care and make the right choices have a very good chance of having healthy babies.

Prenatal Care

See a doctor as soon as possible after you find out you're pregnant to begin getting prenatal care (medical care during pregnancy). The sooner you start to get medical care, the better your chances that you and your baby will be healthy.

If you can't afford to go to a doctor or clinic for prenatal care, social service organizations can help you. Ask your parent, school counselor, or another trusted adult to help you locate resources in your community.

During your first visit, the doctor will ask you lots of questions, including the date of your last period. This helps the doctor estimate how long you have been pregnant and your due date.

Doctors measure pregnancies in weeks. A baby's due date is only an estimate, though: Most babies are born between 38 and 42 weeks after the first day of a woman's last menstrual period, or 36 to 40 weeks after conception (when the sperm fertilizes the egg). Only a small percentage of women actually deliver exactly on their due dates.

About This Chapter: Information in this chapter is from "Having A Healthy Pregnancy," January 2008, reprinted with permission from www.kidshealth.org. Copyright © 2008 The Nemours Foundation. This information was provided by KidsHealth, one of the largest resources online for medically reviewed health information written for parents, kids, and teens. For more articles like this one, visit www.KidsHealth.org, or www.TeensHealth.org.

Timelines

A pregnancy is divided into three phases, or trimesters. The first trimester is from conception to the end of week 13. The second trimester is from week 14 to the end of week 26. The third trimester is from week 27 to the end of the pregnancy.

The doctor will examine you and perform a pelvic exam. He or she may also perform blood tests, a urine test, and tests for sexually transmitted diseases (STDs), including a test for human immunodeficiency virus (HIV), which is on the rise in teens. (Some STDs can cause serious medical problems in newborns, so it's important to get treatment to protect the baby.)

The doctor will explain the types of physical and emotional changes you can expect during pregnancy. He or she will also teach you to how to recognize the signs of possible problems during pregnancy (called complications). This is especially important because teens are more at risk for certain complications, such as anemia, high blood pressure, and delivering a baby earlier than usual (called premature delivery).

Ideally, you should see your doctor once each month for the first 28 weeks of your pregnancy, then every two weeks until 36 weeks, then once a week until you deliver the baby. If you have a medical condition such as diabetes that needs careful monitoring during your pregnancy, your doctor will probably want to see you more often.

It's A Fact!

Your doctor will want you to start taking prenatal vitamins that contain folic acid, calcium, and iron as soon as possible. The doctor may prescribe the vitamins or recommend a brand that you can buy over the counter. These vitamins and minerals help ensure the baby's and mother's health as well as prevent some types of birth defects.

During visits, your doctor will check your weight, blood pressure, and urine, and will measure your abdomen to keep track of the baby's growth. Once the baby's heartbeat can be heard with a special device, the doctor will listen for it at each visit. Your doctor will probably also send you for some other tests during the pregnancy, such as an ultrasound, to make sure that everything is OK with your baby.

One part of prenatal care is attending classes where expectant mothers can learn about having a healthy pregnancy and delivery and the basics of caring for a new baby. These classes may be offered at hospitals, medical centers, schools, and colleges in your area.

It can be difficult for adults to talk to their doctors about their bodies and even more diffi-cult for teens to do so. Your doctor is there to help you stay healthy during pregnancy and have a healthy baby—and there's probably not much he or she hasn't heard from expectant mothers! So don't be afraid to ask questions.

Be upfront when your doctor asks questions, even if they seem embarrassing. A lot of the issues the doctor brings up could affect your baby's health. Think of your doctor both as a re-source and a friend who you can confide in about what's happening to you.

Changes To Expect In Your Body

Pregnancy causes lots of physical changes in the body. Here are some common ones:

Breast Growth

An increase in breast size is one of the first signs of pregnancy, and the breasts may con-tinue to grow throughout the pregnancy. You may go up several bra sizes during the course of your pregnancy.

Skin Changes

Don't be surprised if people tell you your skin is "glowing" when you are pregnant—pregnancy causes an increase in blood volume, which can make your cheeks a little pinker than usual. And hormonal changes increase oil gland secretion, which can give your skin a shinier appearance. Acne is also common during pregnancy for the same reason.

Other skin changes caused by pregnancy hormones may include brownish or yellowish patches on the face called chloasma and a dark line on the midline of the lower abdomen, known as the linea nigra.

Also, moles or freckles that you had prior to pregnancy may become bigger and darker. Even the areola, the area around the nipples, becomes darker. Stretch marks are thin pink or purplish lines that can appear on your abdomen, breasts, or thighs.

Except for the darkening of the areola, which can last, these skin changes will usually dis-appear after you give birth.

Mood Swings

It's very common to have mood swings during pregnancy. Some girls may also experience depression during pregnancy or after delivery. If you have symptoms of depression such as sadness, changes in sleep patterns, thoughts of hurting yourself, or bad feelings about yourself or your life, tell your doctor so he or she can help you to get treatment.

Pregnancy Discomforts

Pregnancy can cause some uncomfortable side effects. These include:

- nausea and vomiting (especially early in the pregnancy)
- leg swelling
- varicose veins in the legs and the area around the vaginal opening
- hemorrhoids
- heartburn and constipation
- backache
- fatigue
- sleep loss

> ### Quick Tip
> If you are pregnant and have bleeding or pain, call the doctor immediately, even if you are not planning to continue the pregnancy.

If you have one or more of these side effects, keep in mind that you're not alone! Ask your doctor for advice on how to deal with these common problems.

Things To Avoid

Smoking, drinking alcohol, and taking drugs when you are pregnant put you and your baby at risk for a number of serious problems.

Alcohol

Doctors now believe that it's not safe to drink any amount of alcohol when you are pregnant. Drinking can harm a developing fetus, putting a baby at risk for birth defects and mental problems.

Smoking

The risks of smoking during pregnancy include stillbirths (when a baby dies while inside the mother), low birth weight (which increases a baby's risk for health problems), prematurity (when babies are born earlier than 37 weeks), and sudden infant death syndrome (SIDS). SIDS is the sudden, unexplained death of an infant who is younger than one year old.

Drugs

Using illegal drugs such as cocaine or marijuana during pregnancy can cause miscarriage, prematurity, and other medical problems. Babies can also be born addicted to certain drugs.

Unsafe Sex

Talk to your doctor about sex during pregnancy. If your doctor says it's OK to have sex while you're pregnant, you must use a condom to help prevent getting an STD. Some STDs can cause blindness, pneumonia, or meningitis in newborns, so it's important to protect yourself and your baby.

Quick Tip

Ask your doctor for help if you are having trouble quitting smoking, drinking, or drugs. Check with your doctor before taking any medication while you are pregnant, including over-the-counter medications, herbal remedies and supplements, and vitamins.

Taking Care Of Yourself During Pregnancy

Eating

Many girls worry about how their bodies look and are afraid to gain weight during pregnancy. But now that you are eating for two, this is not a good time to cut calories or go on a diet. Both you and your baby need certain nutrients so the baby can grow properly. Eating a variety of healthy foods, drinking plenty of water, and cutting back on high-fat junk foods will help you and your developing baby to be healthy.

Doctors generally recommend adding about 300 calories a day to your diet to provide adequate nourishment for the developing fetus. You should gain about 25 to 35 pounds during pregnancy, most of this during the last six months—although how much a girl should gain depends on how much she weighed before the pregnancy. Your doctor will advise you based on your individual situation.

Eating additional fiber—25 to 30 grams a day—and drinking plenty of water can help to prevent common problems such as constipation. Good sources of fiber are fresh fruits and vegetables and breads, cereals, or muffins that have lots of whole grain in them.

You'll need to avoid eating or drinking certain things during pregnancy, such as:

- certain types of fish, such as swordfish, canned tuna, and other fish that may be high in mercury (your doctor can help you decide which fish you can eat)

- foods that contain raw eggs, such as mousse or Caesar salad

- raw or undercooked meat and fish

- processed meats, such as hot dogs and deli meats

- soft, unpasteurized cheeses, such as feta, brie, blue, and goat cheese

- unpasteurized milk, juice, or cider

It's also a good idea to limit artificial sweeteners, and drinks that contain caffeine and artificial sweeteners.

Exercise

Exercising during pregnancy is good for you as long as you are having an uncomplicated pregnancy and choose appropriate activities. Doctors generally recommend low-impact activities such as walking, swimming, and yoga. Contact sports and high-impact aerobic activities that pose a greater risk of injury should generally be avoided. Also, working at a job that involves heavy lifting is not recommended for women during pregnancy. Talk to your doctor if you have questions about whether particular types of exercise are safe for you and your baby.

Sleep

It's important to get plenty of rest while you are pregnant. Early in your pregnancy, try to get into the habit of sleeping on your side. Lying on your side with your knees bent is likely to be the most comfortable position as your pregnancy progresses. Also, it makes your heart's job easier because it keeps the baby's weight from applying pressure to the large vein that carries blood back to the heart from your feet and legs.

Some doctors recommend that girls who are pregnant sleep on the left side. Because of where some of your major blood vessels are, lying on your left side helps keep the uterus from pressing on them. Ask what your doctor recommends—in most cases, lying on either side should do the trick and help take some pressure off your back.

Throughout your pregnancy, but especially toward the end, you may wake up often at night to go to the bathroom. While it's important to drink enough water while you're pregnant, try to drink most of it during the day rather than at night. Use the bathroom right before going to bed. As you get further along in your pregnancy, you might have a difficult time getting comfortable in bed. Try positioning pillows around and under your belly, back, or legs to get more comfortable.

Stress can also interfere with sleep. Maybe you're worried about your baby's health, about delivery, or about what your new role as a parent will be like. All of these feelings are normal, but they may keep you up at night. Talk to your doctor if you are having problems sleeping during your pregnancy.

Emotional Health

It's common for pregnant teens to feel a range of emotions, such as fear, anger, guilt, confusion, and sadness. It may take a while to adjust to the fact that you're going to have a baby. It's a huge change, and it's natural for pregnant teens to wonder whether they're ready to handle the responsibilities that come with being a parent.

How a girl feels often depends on how much support she has from the baby's father, from her family (and the baby's father's family), and from friends. Each girl's situation is different. Depending on your situation, you may need to seek more support from people outside your family. It's important to talk to the people who can support and guide you and help you share and sort through your feelings. Your school counselor or nurse can refer you to resources in your community that can help.

It's A Fact!

Sometimes girls who are pregnant have miscarriages and lose the pregnancy. This can be very upsetting and difficult to go through for some girls, although it may bring feelings of relief for others. It is important to talk about these feelings and to get support from friends and family— or if that's not possible, from people such as counselors or teachers.

School And The Future

Some girls plan to raise their babies themselves. Sometimes grandparents or other family members help. Some girls decide to give their babies up for adoption. It takes a great deal of courage and concern for the baby to make these difficult decisions.

Girls who complete high school are more likely to have good jobs and enjoy more success in their lives. If possible, finish high school now rather than trying to return later. Ask your school counselor or an adult you trust for information about programs and classes in your community for pregnant teens.

Some communities have support groups especially for teen parents. Some high schools have child-care centers on campus. Perhaps a family member or friend can care for your baby while you're in school.

You can learn more about what to expect in becoming a parent by reading books, attending classes, or checking out reputable websites on child raising. Your baby's doctor, your parents, family members, or other adults can all help guide you while you are pregnant and after the baby is born.

Chapter 14

Prenatal Care And Tests

Medical checkups and screening tests help keep you and your baby healthy during pregnancy. This is called prenatal care. It also involves education and counseling about how to handle different aspects of your pregnancy. During your visits, your doctor may discuss many issues, such as healthy eating and physical activity, screening tests you might need, and what to expect during labor and delivery.

Choosing A Prenatal Care Provider

You will see your prenatal care provider many times before you have your baby. So you want to be sure that the person you choose has a good reputation and listens to and respects you. You will want to find out if the doctor or midwife can deliver your baby in the place you want to give birth, such as a specific hospital or birthing center. Your provider also should be willing and able to give you the information and support you need to make an informed choice about whether to breastfeed or bottle-feed.

Health care providers that care for women during pregnancy include the following:

- Obstetricians (OBs) are medical doctors who specialize in the care of pregnant women and in delivering babies. OBs also have special training in surgery so they are also able to do a cesarean delivery. Women who have health problems or are at risk for pregnancy complications should see an obstetrician. Women with the highest risk pregnancies might need special care from a maternal-fetal medicine specialist.

About This Chapter: Information in this chapter is from "Prenatal Care and Tests," a publication of the Office on Women's Health, U.S. Department of Health and Human Services, September 2010.

- Family practice doctors are medical doctors who provide care for the whole family through all stages of life. This includes care during pregnancy and delivery, and following birth. Most family practice doctors cannot perform cesarean deliveries.

- A certified nurse-midwife (CNM) and certified professional midwife (CPM) are trained to provide pregnancy and postpartum care. Midwives can be a good option for healthy women at low risk for problems during pregnancy, labor, or delivery. A CNM is educated in both nursing and midwifery. Most CNMs practice in hospitals and birth centers. A CPM is required to have experience delivering babies in home settings because most CPMs practice in homes and birthing centers. All midwives should have a backup plan with an obstetrician in case of a problem or emergency.

Ask your primary care doctor, friends, and family members for provider recommendations.

It's A Fact!

Some hospitals and birth centers have taken special steps to create the best possible environment for successful breastfeeding. They are called Baby-Friendly Hospitals and Birth Centers. Women who deliver in a baby-friendly facility are promised the information and support they need to breastfeed their infants.

Places To Deliver Your Baby

Many women have strong views about where and how they'd like to deliver their babies. In general, women can choose to deliver at a hospital, birth center, or at home. You will need to contact your health insurance provider to find out what options are available. Also, find out if the doctor or midwife you are considering can deliver your baby in the place you want to give birth.

Hospitals are a good choice for women with health problems or pregnancy complications, or those who are at risk for problems during labor and delivery. Hospitals offer the most advanced medical equipment and highly trained doctors for pregnant women and their babies. In a hospital, doctors can do a cesarean delivery if you or your baby is in danger during labor. Women can get epidurals or many other pain relief options. Also, more and more hospitals now offer onsite birth centers, which aim to offer a style of care similar to standalone birth centers.

Birth or birthing centers give women a homey environment in which to labor and give birth. They try to make labor and delivery a natural and personal process by doing away with most high-tech equipment and routine procedures. So, you will not automatically be hooked up to an IV. Likewise, you won't have an electronic fetal monitor around your belly the whole time. Instead, the midwife or nurse will check in on your baby from time to time with a handheld machine. Once the baby is born, all exams and care will occur in your room. Usually certified nurse-midwives, not obstetricians, deliver babies at birth centers. Healthy women who are at low risk for problems during pregnancy, labor, and delivery may choose to deliver at a birth center.

Many birthing centers have showers or tubs in their rooms for laboring women. They also tend to have comforts of home like large beds and rocking chairs. In general, birth centers allow more people in the delivery room than do hospitals.

Birth centers can be inside of hospitals, a part of a hospital, or completely separate facilities. If you want to deliver at a birth center, make sure it meets the standards of the Accreditation Association for Ambulatory Health Care, The Joint Commission, or the American Association of Birth Centers. Accredited birth centers must have doctors who can work at a nearby hospital in case of problems with the mom or baby. Also, make sure the birth center has the staff and setup to support successful breastfeeding.

It's A Fact!

Women cannot receive epidurals at a birth center, although some pain medicines may be available. If a cesarean delivery becomes necessary, women must be moved to a hospital for the procedure. After delivery, babies with problems can receive basic emergency care while being moved to a hospital.

Prenatal Checkups

During pregnancy, regular checkups are very important. This consistent care can help keep you and your baby healthy, spot problems if they occur, and prevent problems during delivery. Typically, routine checkups occur:

- Once each month for weeks four through 28

- Twice a month for weeks 28 through 36

- Weekly for weeks 36 to birth

At your first visit your doctor will perform a full physical exam, take your blood for lab tests, and calculate your due date. Your doctor might also do a breast exam, a pelvic exam to check your uterus (womb), and a cervical exam, including a Pap test. During this first visit, your doctor will ask you lots of questions about your lifestyle, relationships, and health habits. It's important to be honest with your doctor.

After the first visit, most prenatal visits will include:

- Checking your blood pressure and weight

- Checking the baby's heart rate

- Measuring your abdomen to check your baby's growth

You also will have some routine tests throughout your pregnancy, such as tests to look for anemia, tests to measure risk of gestational diabetes, and tests to look for harmful infections.

It's A Fact!

Women with high-risk pregnancies need to see their doctors more often than women who do not have high-risk pregnancies.

Monitor Your Baby's Activity

After 28 weeks, keep track of your baby's movement. This will help you to notice if your baby is moving less than normal, which could be a sign that your baby is in distress and needs a doctor's care. An easy way to do this is the "count to 10" approach. Count your baby's movements in the evening—the time of day when the fetus tends to be most active. Lie down if you have trouble feeling your baby move. Most women count 10 movements within about 20 minutes. But it is rare for a woman to count less than 10 movements within two hours at times when the baby is active. Count your baby's movements every day so you know what is normal for you. Call your doctor if you count less than 10 movements within two hours or if you notice your baby is moving less than normal. If your baby is not moving at all, call your doctor right away.

Quick Tip

Become a partner with your doctor to manage your care. Keep all of your appointments—every one is important! Ask questions and read to educate yourself about this exciting time.

Prenatal Tests

Tests are used during pregnancy to check your and your baby's health. At your fist prenatal visit, your doctor will use tests to check for a number of things, such as the following:

- Your blood type and Rh factor

- Anemia

- Infections, such as toxoplasmosis and sexually transmitted infections (STIs), including hepatitis B, syphilis, chlamydia, and human immunodeficiency virus (HIV)

- Signs that you are immune to rubella (German measles) and chicken pox

Throughout your pregnancy, your doctor or midwife may suggest a number of other tests, too. Some tests are suggested for all women, such as screenings for gestational diabetes, Down syndrome, and HIV. Other tests might be offered based on the following characteristics:

- Age

- Personal or family health history

- Ethnic background

- Results of routine tests

Some tests are screening tests. They detect risks for or signs of possible health problems in you or your baby. Based on screening test results, your doctor might suggest diagnostic tests. Diagnostic tests confirm or rule out health problems in you or your baby.

Common Prenatal Tests

Amniocentesis: This test can diagnosis certain birth defects, including Down syndrome, cystic fibrosis, and spina bifida. It is performed at 14 to 20 weeks. It may be suggested for couples at higher risk for genetic disorders. It also provides DNA for paternity testing.

Avoid Keepsake Ultrasounds

You might think a keepsake ultrasound is a must-have for your scrapbook. But, doctors advise against ultrasound when there is no medical need to do so. Some companies sell keepsake ultrasound videos and images. Although ultrasound is considered safe for medical purposes, exposure to ultrasound energy for a keepsake video or image may put a mother and her unborn baby at risk. Don't take that chance.

A thin needle is used to draw out a small amount of amniotic fluid and cells from the sac surrounding the fetus. The sample is sent to a lab for testing.

Biophysical Profile (BPP): This test is used in the third trimester to monitor the overall health of the baby and to help decide if the baby should be delivered early. BPP involves an ultrasound exam along with a nonstress test. The BPP looks at the baby's breathing, movement, muscle tone, heart rate, and the amount of amniotic fluid.

Chorionic Villus Sampling (CVS): A test done at 10 to 13 weeks to diagnose certain birth defects, including chromosomal disorders such as Down syndrome and genetic disorders such as cystic fibrosis. CVS may be suggested for couples at higher risk for genetic disorders. It also provides DNA for paternity testing. During this test, a needle removes a small sample of cells from the placenta to be tested.

First Trimester Screen: A screening test done at 11 to 14 weeks to detect higher risk of chromosomal disorders, including Down syndrome and trisomy 18, and other problems such as heart defects. It also can reveal multiple births. Based on test results, your doctor may suggest other tests to diagnose a disorder.

Glucose Challenge Screening: A screening test done at 26 to 28 weeks to determine the mother's risk of gestational diabetes. Based on test results, your doctor may suggest a glucose tolerance test. First, you consume a special sugary drink from your doctor. A blood sample is taken one hour later to look for high blood sugar levels.

Glucose Tolerance Test: This test is done at 26 to 28 weeks to diagnose gestational diabetes. Your doctor will tell you what to eat a few days before the test. Then, you cannot eat or drink anything but sips of water for 14 hours before the test. Your blood is drawn to test your fasting blood glucose level. Then, you will consume a sugary drink. Your blood will be tested every hour for three hours to see how well your body processes sugar.

Group B Streptococcus Infection: This test is done at 36 to 37 weeks to look for bacteria that can cause pneumonia or serious infection in a newborn. A swab is used to take cells from your vagina and rectum to be tested.

Maternal Serum Screen: This test is also called quad screen, triple test, triple screen, multiple marker screen, or AFP. It is a screening test done at 15 to 20 weeks to detect higher risk of chromosomal disorders, including Down syndrome and trisomy 18, and neural tube defects such as spina bifida. Based on test results, your doctor may suggest other tests to diagnose a disorder. In this test, blood is drawn to measure the levels of certain substances in the mother's blood.

Nonstress Test (NST): This test is performed after 28 weeks to monitor your baby's health. It can show signs of fetal distress, such as your baby not getting enough oxygen. A belt is placed around the mother's belly to measure the baby's heart rate in response to its own movements.

Ultrasound Exam: An ultrasound exam can be performed at any point during the pregnancy. Ultrasound exams are not routine. But it is not uncommon for women to have a standard ultrasound exam between 18 and 20 weeks to look for signs of problems with the baby's organs and body systems and confirm the age of the fetus and proper growth. It also might be able to tell the sex of your baby. Ultrasound exam is also used as part of the first trimester screen and biophysical profile (BPP).

Urine Test: A urine sample can look for signs of health problems, such as a urinary tract infection, diabetes, and preeclampsia. If your doctor suspects a problem, the sample might be sent to a lab for more in-depth testing.

Understanding Prenatal Tests And Test Results

If your doctor suggests certain prenatal tests, don't be afraid to ask lots of questions. Learning about the test, why your doctor is suggesting it for you, and what the test results could mean can help you cope with any worries or fears you might have. Keep in mind that screening tests do not diagnose problems. They evaluate risk. So if a screening test comes back abnormal, this doesn't mean there is a problem with your baby. More information is needed. Your doctor can explain what test results mean and possible next steps.

High-Risk Pregnancy

Pregnancies with a greater chance of complications are called high risk. But this doesn't mean there will be problems. The following factors may increase the risk of problems during pregnancy:

- Very young age or older than 35

- Overweight or underweight

- Problems in previous pregnancy

- Health conditions you have before you become pregnant, such as high blood pressure, diabetes, autoimmune disorders, cancer, and HIV

- Pregnancy with twins or other multiples

Health problems also may develop during a pregnancy that make it high risk, such as gestational diabetes or preeclampsia. For more information about high-risk pregnancies, see Chapter 30.

Paying For Prenatal Care

Pregnancy can be stressful if you are worried about affording health care for you and your unborn baby. For many women, the extra expenses of prenatal care and preparing for the new baby are overwhelming. The good news is that women in every state can get help to pay for medical care during their pregnancies. Every state in the United States has a program to help. Programs give medical care, information, advice, and other services important for a healthy pregnancy.

To find out about the program in your state, you can do the following:

- Call 800-311-BABY (800-311-2229). This toll-free telephone number will connect you to the Health Department in your area code.

- Call 800-504-7081 for information in Spanish.

- Call or contact your local Health Department.

You may also find help through these places:

- **Local Hospital Or Social Service Agencies:** Ask to speak with a social worker on staff. She or he will be able to tell you where to go for help.

- **Community Clinics:** Some areas have free clinics or clinics that provide free care to women in need.

- **Women, Infants And Children (WIC) Program:** This government program is available in every state. It provides help with food, nutritional counseling, and access to health services for women, infants, and children.

- **Places Of Worship**

It's a Fact!

The Affordable Care Act offers pregnant women more protections and options. Learn more from healthcare.gov.

Chapter 15

Taking Vitamins With Folic Acid During Pregnancy

Why can't I wait until I'm pregnant or planning to get pregnant to start taking folic acid?

Birth defects of the brain and spine (anencephaly and spina bifida) happen in the first few weeks of pregnancy; often before you find out you're pregnant. By the time you realize you're pregnant, it might be too late to prevent those birth defects. Also, half of all pregnancies in the United States are unplanned.

These are two reasons why it is important for all women who can get pregnant to be sure to get 400 micrograms (mcg) of folic acid every day, even if they aren't planning a pregnancy any time soon.

I'm planning to get pregnant this month. Is it too late to start taking folic acid?

The Centers for Disease Control and Prevention (CDC) recommends women take 400 mcg of folic acid every day, starting at least one month before getting pregnant. If you are trying to get pregnant this month, or planning to get pregnant soon, start taking 400 mcg of folic acid today.

I already have a child with spina bifida. Should I do anything different to prepare for my next pregnancy?

Women who had one pregnancy affected by a birth defect of the brain or spine might have another. Talk to your doctor about taking 4,000 micrograms (4.0 milligrams) of folic acid each

About This Chapter: Information in this chapter is from "Folic Acid Questions and Answers," a publication of the Centers for Disease Control and Prevention, March 2011.

day at least one month before getting pregnant and during the first few months of being pregnant. This is ten times the amount most people take. Your doctor will give you a prescription. You should not take more than one multivitamin each day. Taking more than one each day over time could be harmful to you and your baby.

Can't I get enough folic acid by eating a well-balanced healthy diet?

It is hard to eat a diet that has all the nutrients you need every day. Even with careful planning, you might not get all the vitamins you need from your diet alone. That's why it's important to take a vitamin with folic acid every day.

I can't swallow large pills. How can I take a vitamin with folic acid?

These days, multivitamins with folic acid come in chewable chocolate or fruit flavors, liquids, and large oval or smaller round pills.

A single serving of many breakfast cereals also has the amount of folic acid that a woman needs each day. Check the label. Look for cereals that have 100 percent daily value (DV) of folic acid in a serving, which is 400 micrograms (mcg).

Vitamins cost too much. How can I get the vitamin with folic acid that I need?

Many stores offer a single folic acid supplement for just pennies a day. Another good choice is a store brand multivitamin, which includes more of the vitamins a woman needs each day. Unless your doctor suggests a special type, you do not have to choose among vitamins for women or active people. A basic multivitamin meets the needs of most women.

How can I remember to take a vitamin with folic acid every day?

Make it easy to remember by taking your vitamin at the same time every day. Try taking your vitamin when you do one of the following:

- Brush your teeth
- Eat breakfast
- Finish your shower
- Brush your hair

Seeing the vitamin bottle on the bathroom or kitchen counter can help you remember it, too. If you use a cell phone or PDA, you can program it to give you a daily reminder. If you have children, you can take your vitamin when they take theirs.

Today's woman is busy. You know that you should exercise, eat right, and get enough sleep. You might wonder how you can fit another thing into your day. But it only takes a few seconds to take a vitamin to get all the folic acid you need.

Are there other health benefits of taking folic acid?

Folic acid might help to prevent some other birth defects, such as cleft lip and palate and some heart defects. There might also be other health benefits of taking folic acid for both women and men. More research is needed to confirm these other health benefits. All adults should take 400 micrograms (mcg) of folic acid every day.

Is it better to take more than 400 mcg of folic acid every day?

When taking supplements, more is not better. Women who can get pregnant (whether planning to or not) need just 400 mcg of folic acid daily, and they can get this amount from vitamins or fortified foods. This is in addition to eating foods rich in folate. But, your doctor might ask you to take more for certain reasons.

What is folate and how is it different from folic acid?

Folate is a form of the B vitamin folic acid. Folate is found naturally in some foods, such as leafy, dark green vegetables, citrus fruits and juices, and beans.

The body does not use folate as easily as folic acid. We cannot be sure that eating folate would have the same benefits as getting 400 micrograms of manmade (synthetic) folic acid. Women who can get pregnant should consume 400 micrograms of synthetic folic acid in addition to the natural food folate from a varied diet.

What is synthetic folic acid?

Synthetic folic acid is the simple, manmade form of the B vitamin folate. Folic acid is found in most multivitamins and has been added in U.S. foods labeled as enriched such as bread, pasta, rice, and breakfast cereals. The words folic acid and synthetic folic acid mean the same thing.

Chapter 16

The Stages Of Pregnancy

Pregnancy lasts about 40 weeks, counting from the first day of your last normal period. The weeks are grouped into three trimesters. Find out what's happening with you and your baby in these three stages.

First Trimester (Week 1–Week 12)

During the first trimester your body undergoes many changes. Hormonal changes affect almost every organ system in your body. These changes can trigger symptoms even in the very first weeks of pregnancy. Your period stopping is a clear sign that you are pregnant. Other changes may include the following:

- Extreme tiredness

- Tender, swollen breasts. Your nipples might also stick out.

- Upset stomach with or without throwing up (morning sickness)

- Cravings or distaste for certain foods

- Mood swings

- Constipation (trouble having bowel movements)

- Need to pass urine more often

- Headache

- Heartburn

About This Chapter: Information in this chapter is from "Stages of Pregnancy," a publication of the Office on Women's Health, U.S. Department of Health and Human Services, Sept. 2010.

- Weight gain or loss

As your body changes, you might need to make changes to your daily routine, such as going to bed earlier or eating frequent, small meals. Fortunately, most of these discomforts will go away as your pregnancy progresses. And some women might not feel any discomfort at all. If you have been pregnant before, you might feel differently this time around. Just as each woman is different, so is each pregnancy.

Quick Tip

For some women, body image is a huge concern during pregnancy. Learn what you can do to accept and love your pregnant body at http://www.womenshealth.gov/bodyimage/pregnancy/.

Second Trimester (Week 13–Week 28)

You might notice that symptoms like nausea and fatigue are going away. But other new, more noticeable changes to your body are now happening. Your abdomen will expand as the baby continues to grow. And before this trimester is over, you will feel your baby beginning to move.

As your body changes to make room for your growing baby, you may have the following symptoms:

- Body aches, such as back, abdomen, groin, or thigh pain
- Stretch marks on your abdomen, breasts, thighs, or buttocks
- Darkening of the skin around your nipples
- A line on the skin running from belly button to pubic hairline
- Patches of darker skin, usually over the cheeks, forehead, nose, or upper lip. Patches often match on both sides of the face. This is sometimes called the mask of pregnancy.
- Numb or tingling hands, called carpal tunnel syndrome
- Itching on the abdomen, palms, and soles of the feet. (Call your doctor if you have nausea, loss of appetite, vomiting, jaundice, or fatigue combined with itching. These can be signs of a serious liver problem.)
- Swelling of the ankles, fingers, and face. (If you notice any sudden or extreme swelling or if you gain a lot of weight really quickly, call your doctor right away. This could be a sign of preeclampsia.)

Third Trimester (Week 29–Week 40)

You're in the home stretch. Some of the same discomforts you had in your second trimester will continue. Plus, many women find breathing difficult and notice they have to go to the bathroom even more often. This is because the baby is getting bigger and it is putting more pressure on your organs. Don't worry, your baby is fine and these problems will lessen once you give birth.

Some new body changes you might notice in the third trimester include the following:

- Shortness of breath

- Heartburn

- Swelling of the ankles, fingers, and face. (If you notice any sudden or extreme swelling or if you gain a lot of weight really quickly, call your doctor right away. This could be a sign of preeclampsia.)

- Hemorrhoids

- Tender breasts, which may leak a watery premilk called colostrum

- Your belly button may stick out

- Trouble sleeping

- The baby dropping, or moving lower in your abdomen

- Contractions, which can be a sign of real or false labor

It's A Fact!
You can do something about common pregnancy discomforts. Learn more in Chapter 17.

As you near your due date, your cervix becomes thinner and softer (called effacing). This is a normal, natural process that helps the birth canal (vagina) to open during the birthing process. Your doctor will check your progress with a vaginal exam as you near your due date.

Chapter 17

The Physical Changes And Discomforts Of Pregnancy

Everyone expects pregnancy to bring an expanding waistline. But many women are surprised by the other body changes that pop up. Get the lowdown on stretch marks, weight gain, heartburn, and other joys of pregnancy. Find out what you can do to feel better.

Body Aches

As your uterus expands, you may feel aches and pains in the back, abdomen, groin area, and thighs. Many women also have backaches and aching near the pelvic bone due to the pressure of the baby's head, increased weight, and loosening joints. Some pregnant women complain of pain that runs from the lower back, down the back of one leg, to the knee or foot. This is called sciatica. It is thought to occur when the uterus puts pressure on the sciatic nerve. To relieve these symptoms, rest and apply heat. Call the doctor if the pain does not get better.

Breast Changes

A woman's breasts increase in size and fullness during pregnancy. As the due date approaches, hormone changes will cause your breasts to get even bigger to prepare for breastfeeding. Your breasts may feel full, heavy, or tender. Be sure to wear a maternity bra with good support.

In the third trimester, some pregnant women begin to leak colostrum from their breasts. Colostrum is the first milk that your breasts produce for the baby. It is a thick, yellowish fluid containing antibodies that protect newborns from infection. Put pads in your bra to absorb leakage.

About This Chapter: Information in this chapter is from "Body Changes and Discomforts," a publication of the Office on Women's Health, U.S. Department of Health and Human Services, September 2010.

> **Quick Tip**
> Tell your doctor if you feel a lump or have nipple changes or discharge (that is not colostrum) or skin changes.

Constipation

Many pregnant women complain of constipation. Signs of constipation include having hard, dry stools; fewer than three bowel movements per week; and painful bowel movements. Higher levels of hormones due to pregnancy slow down digestion and relax muscles in the bowels leaving many women constipated. Plus, the pressure of the expanding uterus on the bowels can contribute to constipation.

To relieve constipation, do the following:

- Drink eight to 10 glasses of water daily.

- Don't drink caffeine.

- Eat fiber-rich foods, such as fresh or dried fruit, raw vegetables, and whole-grain cereals and breads.

- Try mild physical activity.

- Tell your doctor if constipation does not go away.

Dizziness

Many pregnant women complain of dizziness and lightheadedness throughout their pregnancies. Fainting is rare but does happen even in some healthy pregnant women. If you are feeling dizzy, the following steps may help: stand up slowly; avoid standing for too long; don't skip meals; lie on your left side; wear loose clothing. Call the doctor if you feel faint and have vaginal bleeding or abdominal pain.

Fatigue And Sleep Problems

During your pregnancy, you might feel tired even after you've had a lot of sleep. Many women find they're exhausted in the first trimester. Don't worry, this is normal. This is your body's way of telling you that you need more rest. In the second trimester, tiredness is usually replaced with a feeling of well being and energy. But in the third trimester, exhaustion often sets in again. As you get larger, sleeping may become more difficult. The baby's movements, bathroom runs, and an increase in the body's metabolism might interrupt or disturb your sleep. Leg cramping can also interfere with a good night's sleep. If you are having trouble sleeping, try the following:

- Lie on your left side.
- Use pillows for support, such as behind your back, tucked between your knees, and under your tummy.
- Practice good sleep habits, such as going to bed and getting up at the same time each day and using your bed only for sleep and sex.
- Go to bed a little earlier.
- Nap if you are not able to get enough sleep at night.
- Drink needed fluids earlier in the day, so you can drink less in the hours before bed.

Heartburn And Indigestion

Hormones and the pressure of the growing uterus cause indigestion and heartburn. Try these tips:

- Eat several small meals instead of three large meals—eat slowly.
- Drink fluids between meals—not with meals.
- Don't eat greasy and fried foods.
- Avoid citrus fruits or juices and spicy foods.
- Do not eat or drink within a few hours of bedtime.
- Do not lie down right after meals.

If symptoms don't improve after trying these suggestions, call your doctor and ask about using an antacid.

Hemorrhoids

Hemorrhoids are swollen and bulging veins in the rectum. They can cause itching, pain, and bleeding. Up to 50 percent of pregnant women get hemorrhoids. To reduce hemorrhoids: drink lots of fluids; eat fiber-rich foods, like whole grains, raw or cooked leafy green vegetables, and fruits; and try not to strain with bowel movements.

> **Quick Tip**
>
> Talk to your doctor about using products such as witch hazel to soothe hemorrhoids.

Itching

About 20 percent of pregnant women feel itchy during pregnancy. Usually women feel itchy in the abdomen. But red, itchy palms and soles of the feet are also common complaints. To reduce itching: use gentle soaps and moisturizing creams; avoid hot showers and baths; and avoid itchy fabrics. Call your doctor if symptoms don't improve after a week of self-care.

Leg Cramps

At different times during your pregnancy, you might have sudden muscle spasms in your legs or feet. They usually occur at night. This is due to a change in the way your body processes calcium. To reduce leg cramps, gently stretch muscles and get mild exercise. For sudden cramps, flex your foot forward. Eat calcium-rich foods. Ask your doctor about calcium supplements.

Morning Sickness

In the first trimester hormone changes can cause nausea and vomiting. This is called morning sickness, although it can occur at any time of day. Morning sickness usually tapers off by the second trimester. Try these tips:

- Eat several small meals instead of three large meals to keep your stomach from being empty.

- Don't lie down after meals.

- Eat dry toast, saltines, or dry cereals before getting out of bed in the morning.

- Eat bland foods that are low in fat and easy to digest, such as cereal, rice, and bananas.

- Sip on water, weak tea, or clear soft drinks. Or eat ice chips.

- Avoid smells that upset your stomach.

Call your doctor if you have flu-like symptoms, which may signal a more serious condition, or if you have severe, constant nausea and/or vomiting several times every day.

Nasal Problems

Nosebleeds and nasal stuffiness are common during pregnancy. To reduce nasal problems, blow your nose gently, drink fluids, and use a cool mist humidifier. To stop a nosebleed, squeeze your nose between your thumb and forefinger for a few minutes. Call your doctor if nosebleeds are frequent and do not stop after a few minutes.

Numb Or Tingling Hands

Feelings of swelling, tingling, and numbness in fingers and hands, called carpal tunnel syndrome, can occur during pregnancy. These symptoms are due to swelling of tissues in the narrow passages in your wrists, and they should disappear after delivery. Take frequent breaks to rest hands. Ask your doctor about fitting you for a splint to keep wrists straight.

Stretch Marks And Skin Changes

Stretch marks are red, pink, or brown streaks on the skin. Most often they appear on the thighs, buttocks, abdomen, and breasts. These scars are caused by the stretching of the skin, and usually appear in the second half of pregnancy.

Some women notice other skin changes during pregnancy. For many women, the nipples become darker and browner during pregnancy. Many pregnant women also develop a dark line (called the linea nigra) on the skin that runs from the belly button down to the pubic hairline. Patches of darker skin usually over the cheeks, forehead, nose, or upper lip also are common. Patches often match on both sides of the face. These spots are called melasma or chloasma and are more common in darker-skinned women.

Swelling

Many women develop mild swelling in the face, hands, or ankles at some point in their pregnancies. As the due date approaches, swelling often becomes more noticeable. To reduce swelling, drink eight to 10 glasses of fluids daily. Don't drink caffeine or eat salty foods. Rest and elevate your feet. Ask your doctor about support hose. Call your doctor if your hands or feet swell suddenly or you rapidly gain weight—it may be preeclampsia.

It's A Fact!
Stretch marks and other changes usually fade after delivery.

Urinary Frequency And Leaking

Temporary bladder control problems are common in pregnancy. Your unborn baby pushes down on the bladder, urethra, and pelvic floor muscles. This pressure can lead to a more frequent need to urinate, as well as leaking of urine when sneezing, coughing, or laughing. Try these tips: take frequent bathroom breaks; drink plenty of fluids to avoid dehydration; and do Kegel exercises to tone pelvic muscles. Call your doctor if you experience burning along with frequency of urination—it may be an infection.

Varicose Veins

During pregnancy blood volume increases greatly. This can cause veins to enlarge. Plus, pressure on the large veins behind the uterus causes the blood to slow in its return to the heart. For these reasons, varicose veins in the legs and anus (hemorrhoids) are more common in pregnancy.

Varicose veins look like swollen veins raised above the surface of the skin. They can be twisted or bulging and are dark purple or blue in color. They are found most often on the backs of the calves or on the inside of the leg. To reduce varicose veins, avoid tight knee-highs and sit with your legs and feet raised.

Chapter 18

Nutrition And Exercise During Pregnancy

A Healthy Eating Plan

A healthy eating plan for pregnancy includes a variety of nutrient-rich foods. The U.S. Department of Health and Human Services and the U.S. Department of Agriculture jointly release *Dietary Guidelines for Americans*. These guidelines, updated every five years, outline recommendations to promote health and reduce the risk of chronic disease through nutritious eating and physical activity. The recommendations include some of the nutritional needs of pregnancy. For more information about food groups and nutrition values, visit: www.healthierus.gov/dietaryguidelines.

Calories

Eating a variety of foods that provide enough calories helps you and your baby gain the proper amount of weight. During the first three months of your pregnancy, you do not need to change the number of calories you get from the foods you eat.

Normal-weight women need an extra 300 calories each day during the last six months of pregnancy. This totals about 1,900 to 2,500 calories a day. If you were underweight, overweight, or obese before you became pregnant, or if you are pregnant with more than one baby, you may need a different number of calories. Talk to your health care provider about how much weight you should gain and how many calories you need.

About This Chapter: Information in this chapter is from "Fit for Two: Tips for Pregnancy," a publication of the National Institute of Diabetes and Digestive and Kidney Diseases (NIDDK), November 2009.

Weight Gain

Gaining a healthy amount of weight may help you have a more comfortable pregnancy and delivery. It also may help you have fewer pregnancy complications, such as diabetes, high blood pressure, constipation, and backaches.

Talk to your health care provider about how much weight you should gain during your pregnancy. General weight-gain recommendations listed below refer to weight before pregnancy and are for women expecting only one baby.

Gaining too little weight during your pregnancy makes it hard for your baby to grow properly. Talk to your health care provider if you feel you are not gaining enough weight.

If you gain too much weight, you may have a longer labor and more difficult delivery. Also, gaining a lot of extra body fat will make it harder for you to return to a healthy weight after you have your baby. If you feel you are gaining too much weight during your pregnancy, talk with your health care provider.

Table 18.1. Weight-Gain Recommendations

If you are:	You should gain:
Underweight	About 28 to 40 pounds
Normal weight	About 25 to 35 pounds
Overweight	About 15 to 25 pounds
Obese	At least 15 pounds

Quick Tip

Do not try to lose weight if you are pregnant. If you do not eat enough calories or a variety of foods, your baby will not get the nutrients he or she needs to grow.

Source: NIDDK, November 2009.

Special Nutritional Needs

During pregnancy, you and your growing baby need more of several nutrients. By eating the recommended number of daily servings from each of the five food groups, you should get most of the nutrients you need.

Be sure to include foods high in folate, such as orange juice, strawberries, spinach, broccoli, beans, and fortified breads and breakfast cereals. Or get it in a vitamin/mineral supplement.

To help prevent birth defects, you must get enough daily folate before as well as during pregnancy. Prenatal supplements contain folic acid (another form of folate). Look for a supplement that has at least 400 micrograms (0.4 milligrams) of folic acid.

> ## It's A Fact!
>
> If you follow a vegetarian diet, you can continue it during your pregnancy, but talk to your health care provider first.
>
> To make sure you are getting enough important nutrients, including protein, iron, vitamin B12, and vitamin D, your health care provider may ask you to meet with a registered dietitian who can help you plan meals. Your health care provider may also recommend that you take supplements.
>
> Source: NIDDK, November 2009.

Although most health care providers recommend taking a multivitamin/mineral prenatal supplement before becoming pregnant, during pregnancy, and while breastfeeding, always talk to your health care provider before taking any supplements.

Tips For Healthy Eating

Meet the needs of your body and help avoid common discomforts of pregnancy by following these tips:

- **Eat breakfast every day.** If you feel sick to your stomach in the morning, choose dry whole-wheat toast or whole-grain crackers when you first wake up—even before you get out of bed. Eat the rest of your breakfast (fruit, oatmeal, cereal, milk, yogurt, or other foods) later in the morning.

- **Eat high-fiber foods.** Eating whole-grain cereals, vegetables, fruits, beans, whole-wheat breads, and brown rice, along with drinking plenty of water and getting daily physical activity, can help you prevent the constipation that many women have during pregnancy.

- **Keep healthy foods on hand.** A fruit bowl filled with apples, bananas, peaches, oranges, and grapes makes it easy to grab a healthy snack. Fresh, frozen, and canned fruits and vegetables make healthy and quick additions to meals, as do canned beans. Be sure to choose canned fruits packed in their own juices. Also, rinse canned beans and vegetables with water before preparing, which helps remove excess salt.

- **If you have heartburn during your pregnancy, eat small meals more often,** eat slowly, avoid spicy and fatty foods (such as hot peppers or fried chicken), drink beverages between meals instead of with meals, and do not lie down soon after eating.

- **If you have morning sickness, or hyperemesis, talk with your health care provider.** You may need to adjust the way you eat and drink, such as by eating smaller meals more frequently and drinking plenty of fluids. Your health care provider can help you deal with morning sickness while keeping your healthy eating habits on track.

It's A Fact!

- DON'T drink raw or unpasteurized milk or juice or eat foods that contain unpasteurized milk.
- DON'T eat unwashed fruits and vegetables.
- DON'T eat raw sprouts of any kind (including alfalfa, clover, radish, and mung bean).

Source: From "Healthy Pregnancy: Food Don'ts," a publication of the Office on Women's Health, U.S. Department of Health and Human Services, September 2010.

Foods To Avoid

There are certain foods and beverages that can harm your baby if you eat or drink them while you are pregnant. Here is a general list of foods and beverages that you should avoid:

- **Alcohol**. Instead of wine, beer, or a mixed drink, enjoy apple cider, tomato juice, sparkling water, or other nonalcoholic beverages.

- **Fish that may have high levels of methyl-mercury (a substance that can build up in fish and harm an unborn baby).** Do not eat shark, swordfish, king mackerel, and tilefish during pregnancy. Eat no more than 12 ounces of any fish per week (equal to four three-ounce servings—each about the size of a deck of cards).

- **Soft cheeses such as feta, Brie, and goat cheese and ready-to-eat meats including lunch meats, hot dogs, and deli meats.** These foods may contain bacteria called listeria that are harmful to unborn babies. Cooking lunch meats, hot dogs, and deli meats until steaming hot can kill the bacteria and make these meats safe to eat.

- **Raw or undercooked fish, meat and poultry.** Avoid raw fish dishes, such as sashimi and some types of sushi and ceviche. When raw or undercooked, these foods may contain harmful bacteria. Cook fish, meat, and poultry thoroughly before eating.

- **Large amounts of caffeine-containing beverages.** If you are a heavy coffee, tea, or soda drinker, talk to your health care provider about whether you should cut back on caffeine. Try a decaffeinated version of your favorite beverage, a mug of warm low-fat or fat-free milk, or sparkling mineral water.

- **Anything that is not food.** Some pregnant women may crave something that is not food, such as laundry starch or clay. Talk to your health care provider if you crave something that is not food.

Quick Tip

Ask your health care provider for a complete list of foods and beverages that you should avoid.

Source: NIDDK, November 2009.

Physical Activity

Almost all women can and should be physically active during pregnancy. Talk to your health care provider first, particularly if you have high blood pressure, diabetes, anemia, bleeding, or other disorders, or if you are obese or underweight.

Whether or not you were active before you were pregnant, ask your health care provider about a level of exercise that is safe for you. Aim to be physically active at a moderate-intensity level (one that makes you breathe harder but does not overwork or overheat you) on most, if not all, days of the week.

Regular, moderate-intensity physical activity during pregnancy may do the following:

- Help you and your baby to gain the proper amounts of weight.

- Reduce the discomforts of pregnancy, such as backaches, leg cramps, constipation, bloating, and swelling.

It's A Fact!

The three main dangers lurking in the food pregnant women eat are the following:

- **Listeria:** A dangerous bacterium that can grow even in cold refrigerators.
- **Mercury:** A harmful metal found in high levels in some fish.
- **Toxoplasma:** A risky parasite found in undercooked meat and unwashed fruits and vegetables.

These things can cause serious illness or even death to you or your unborn baby.

Source: From "Healthy Pregnancy: Food Don'ts," a publication of the Office on Women's Health, U.S. Department of Health and Human Services, September 2010.

- Reduce your risk for gestational diabetes (diabetes found for the first time when a woman is pregnant).

- Improve your mood and energy level.

- Improve your sleep.

- Help you have an easier, shorter labor.

- Help you to recover from delivery and return to a healthy weight faster.

Follow these safety precautions while being active during your pregnancy:

- Choose moderate activities that are unlikely to injure you, such as walking, aqua aerobics, swimming, yoga, or using a stationary bike.

- Stop exercising when you start to feel tired, and never exercise until you are exhausted or overheated.

- Drink plenty of fluids before, during, and after being physically active.

- Wear comfortable clothing that fits well and supports and protects your breasts.

- Stop exercising if you feel dizzy, short of breath, or sick to your stomach. You should also stop if you notice pain in your back, swelling, or numbness, or that your heart is beating too fast or at an uneven rate.

Physical Activities To Avoid

For your health and safety, and for the health of your baby, you should not do certain physical activities while you are pregnant. Some of these are listed below. Talk to your health care provider about other physical activities that you should avoid during your pregnancy.

- Avoid being active outside during hot weather.

- Avoid steam rooms, hot tubs, and saunas.

- Avoid physical activities, such as certain yoga poses, that call for you to lie flat on your back after 20 weeks of pregnancy.

- Avoid contact sports and activities that may cause injury, such as football and boxing, and horseback riding.

- Avoid activities that make you jump or change directions quickly, such as tennis or basketball. During pregnancy, your joints loosen and you are more likely to hurt yourself when doing these activities.

- Avoid activities that can result in a fall, such as in-line skating or downhill skiing.

Tips To Remember

- Talk to your health care provider about how much weight you should gain during your pregnancy.

- Eat foods rich in folate, iron, calcium, and protein, or get these nutrients through a prenatal supplement.

- Talk to your health care provider before taking any supplements.

- Eat breakfast every day.

- Eat high-fiber foods and drink plenty of water to avoid constipation.

- Avoid alcohol, raw or undercooked fish, fish high in mercury, undercooked meat and poultry, soft cheeses, and anything that is not food.

- Aim to be physically active on most, if not all, days of the week during your pregnancy. Talk to your health care provider before you begin if you have not previously been physically active.

- After pregnancy, slowly get back to your routine of regular, moderate-intensity physical activity. Make sure you feel able and your health care provider says it is safe to be physically active.

- Take pleasure in the miracles of pregnancy and birth.

Chapter 19

Eating Disorders During Pregnancy

Eating disorders affect approximately seven million American women each year and tend to peak during childbearing years. Pregnancy is a time when body image concerns are more prevalent, and for those who are struggling with an eating disorder, the nine months of pregnancy can cause disorders to become more serious.

Two of the most common types of eating disorders are anorexia and bulimia. Anorexia involves obsessive dieting or starvation to control weight gain. Bulimia involves binge eating and vomiting or using laxatives to rid the body of excess calories. Both types of eating disorders may negatively affect the reproductive process and pregnancy.

Eating Disorders Affect Fertility

Eating disorders, particularly anorexia, affect fertility by reducing your chances of conceiving. Most women with anorexia do not have menstrual cycles, and approximately 50 percent of women struggling with bulimia do not have regular menstrual cycles. The absence of menstruation is caused by reduced calorie intake, excessive exercise, and/or psychological stress. If a woman is not having regular periods, getting pregnant can be very challenging.

Eating Disorders Affect Pregnancy

Eating disorders affect pregnancy in a number of ways. The following complications are associated with eating disorders during pregnancy:

- Premature labor

- Low birth weight

- Stillbirth or fetal death

- Increased risk of cesarean birth

- Delayed fetal growth

- Respiratory problems

- Gestational diabetes

- Complications during labor

- Depression

- Miscarriage

- Preeclampsia

> **It's A Fact!**
>
> Women with eating disorders have higher rates of postpartum depression and are more likely to have problems with breastfeeding.

Women who are struggling with bulimia will often gain excess weight, which places them at risk for hypertension.

The laxatives, diuretics, and other medications taken may be harmful to the developing baby. These substances take away nutrients and fluids before they are able to feed and nourish the baby. It is possible they may lead to fetal abnormalities as well, particularly if they are used on a regular basis.

Reproductive Recommendations For Women With Eating Disorders

If you are struggling with an eating disorder, getting help to overcome it is the best thing you can do for your reproductive and pregnancy health. The majority of women with eating disorders can have healthy babies if they have normal weight gain throughout pregnancy.

Here are some suggested guidelines for women with eating disorders who are trying to conceive or have discovered that they are pregnant:

Prior To Pregnancy

- Achieve and maintain a healthy weight.

- Avoid purging.

- Consult your health care provider for a pre-conception appointment.

- Meet with a nutritionist and start a healthy pregnancy diet, which may include prenatal vitamins.

- Seek counseling to address your eating disorder and any underlying concerns; seek both individual and group therapy.

During Pregnancy

- Schedule a prenatal visit early in your pregnancy and inform your health care provider that you have been struggling with an eating disorder.

- Strive for healthy weight gain.

- Eat well-balanced meals with all the appropriate nutrients.

- Find a nutritionist who can help you with healthy and appropriate eating.

- Avoid purging.

- Seek counseling to address your eating disorder and any underlying concerns; seek both individual and group therapy.

After Pregnancy

- Continue counseling to improve physical and mental health.

- Inform your safe network (health care provider, spouse, and friends) of your eating disorder and the increased risk of postpartum depression; ask them to be available after the birth.

- Contact a lactation consultant to help with early breastfeeding.

- Find a nutritionist who can help work with you to stay healthy, manage your weight, and invest in your baby.

Chapter 20

Sleeping During Pregnancy

Expectant parents know that it'll be harder to get a good night's sleep after their little one arrives, but who would have guessed that catching enough ZZZs during pregnancy could be so difficult?

Actually, you may sleep more than usual during the first trimester of your pregnancy. It's normal to feel tired as your body works to protect and nurture the developing baby. The placenta (the organ that nourishes the fetus until birth) is just forming, your body is making more blood, and your heart is pumping faster.

Why Sleeping Can Be Difficult

The first and most pressing reason behind sleep problems during pregnancy is the increasing size of the fetus, which can make it hard to find a comfortable sleeping position. If you've always been a back or stomach sleeper, you might have trouble getting used to sleeping on your side (as doctors recommend). Also, shifting around in bed becomes more difficult as the pregnancy progresses and your size increases.

Other common physical symptoms may interfere with sleep as well:

- **The Frequent Urge To Urinate:** Your kidneys are working harder to filter the increased volume of blood (30 percent to 50 percent more than you had before pregnancy) moving through your body, and this filtering process results in more urine. Also, as your baby grows and the uterus gets bigger, the pressure on your bladder increases. This means more trips to the bathroom, day and night. The number of nighttime trips may be greater if your baby is particularly active at night.

- **Increased Heart Rate:** Your heart rate increases during pregnancy to pump more blood, and as more of your blood supply goes to the uterus, your heart will be working harder to send sufficient blood to the rest of your body.

- **Shortness Of Breath:** At first, your breathing may be affected by the increase in pregnancy hormones, which will cause you to breathe in more deeply. This might make you feel as if you're working harder to get air. Later on, breathing can feel more difficult as your enlarging uterus takes up more space, resulting in pressure against your diaphragm (the muscle just below your lungs).

- **Leg Cramps And Backaches:** Pains in your legs or back are caused in part by the extra weight you're carrying. During pregnancy, the body also produces a hormone called relaxin, which helps prepare it for childbirth. One of the effects of relaxin is the loosening of ligaments throughout the body, making pregnant women less stable and more prone to injury, especially in their backs.

- **Heartburn And Constipation:** Many women experience heartburn, which occurs when the stomach contents reflux back up into the esophagus. During pregnancy, the entire digestive system slows down and food tends to remain in the stomach and intestines longer, which may cause heartburn or constipation. These can both get worse later on in the pregnancy when the growing uterus presses on the stomach or the large intestine.

Your sleep problems might have other causes as well. Many pregnant women report that their dreams become more vivid than usual, and some even experience nightmares.

Stress can interfere with sleep, too. Maybe you're worried about your baby's health, anxious about your abilities as a parent, or feeling nervous about the delivery itself. All of these feelings are normal, but they might keep you (and your partner) up at night.

It's A Fact!
It's usually later in pregnancy that most women have trouble getting enough deep, uninterrupted sleep.

Finding A Good Sleeping Position

Early in your pregnancy, try to get into the habit of sleeping on your side. Lying on your side with your knees bent is likely to be the most comfortable position as your pregnancy progresses. It also makes your heart's job easier because it keeps the baby's weight from applying pressure to the large vein (called the inferior vena cava) that carries blood back to the heart from your feet and legs.

Some doctors specifically recommend that pregnant women sleep on the left side. Because your liver is on the right side of your abdomen, lying on your left side helps keep the uterus off that large organ. Sleeping on the left side also improves circulation to the heart and allows for the best blood flow to the fetus, uterus, and kidneys. Ask what your doctor recommends—in most cases, lying on either side should do the trick and help take some pressure off your back.

But don't drive yourself crazy worrying that you might roll over onto your back during the night. Shifting positions is a natural part of sleeping that you can't control. Most likely, during the third trimester of your pregnancy, your body won't shift into the back-sleeping position anyway because it will be too uncomfortable.

If you do shift onto your back and the baby's weight presses on your inferior vena cava, the discomfort will probably wake you up. See what your doctor recommends about this; he or she may suggest that you use a pillow to keep yourself propped up on one side.

Quick Tip

Try experimenting with pillows to discover a comfortable sleeping position. Some women find that it helps to place a pillow under their abdomen or between their legs. Also, using a bunched-up pillow or rolled-up blanket at the small of your back may help to relieve some pressure. In fact, you'll see many pregnancy pillows on the market. If you're thinking about buying one, talk with your doctor first about which might work for you.

Tips For Sleeping Success

Although they might seem appealing when you're feeling desperate to get some ZZZs, remember that over-the-counter sleep aids, including herbal remedies, are not recommended for pregnant women. Instead, these tips may safely improve your chances of getting a good night's sleep:

- Cut out caffeinated drinks like soda, coffee, and tea from your diet as much as possible. Restrict any intake of them to the morning or early afternoon.

- Avoid drinking a lot of fluids or eating a full meal within a few hours of going to bed at night. (But make sure that you also get plenty of nutrients and liquids throughout the day.) Some women find it helpful to eat more at breakfast and lunch and then have a smaller dinner. If nausea is keeping you up, try eating a few crackers before you go to bed.

- Get into a routine of going to bed and waking up at the same time each day.

- Avoid rigorous exercise right before you go to bed. Instead, do something relaxing, like soaking in a warm bath for 15 minutes or having a warm, caffeine-free drink, such as milk with honey or a cup of herbal tea.

- If a leg cramp awakens you, it may help to press your feet hard against the wall or to stand on the leg. Also, make sure that you're getting enough calcium in your diet, which can help reduce leg cramps.

- Take a class in yoga or learn other relaxation techniques to help you unwind after a busy day. (Be sure to discuss any new activity or fitness regimen with your doctor first.)

- If fear and anxiety are keeping you awake, consider enrolling in a childbirth or parenting class. More knowledge and the company of other pregnant women may help to ease the fears that are keeping you awake at night.

When You Can't Sleep

Of course, there are bound to be times when you just can't sleep. Instead of tossing and turning, worrying that you're not asleep, and counting the hours until your alarm clock will go off, get up and do something: read a book, listen to music, watch TV, catch up on letters or e-mail, or pursue some other activity you enjoy. Eventually, you'll probably feel tired enough to get back to sleep.

And if possible, take short naps (30 to 60 minutes) during the day to make up for lost sleep. It won't be long before your baby will be setting the sleep rules in your house, so you might as well get used to sleeping in spurts!

Chapter 21

Depression During And After Pregnancy

What is depression?

Depression is more than just feeling blue or down in the dumps for a few days. It's a serious illness that involves the brain. With depression, sad, anxious, or empty feelings don't go away; instead, they interfere with day-to-day life and routines. These feelings can be mild to severe. The good news is that most people with depression get better with treatment.

How common is depression during and after pregnancy?

Depression is a common problem during and after pregnancy. About 13 percent of pregnant women and new mothers have depression.

How do I know if I have depression?

When you are pregnant or after you have a baby, you may be depressed and not know it. Some normal changes during and after pregnancy can cause symptoms similar to those of depression. But if you have any of the following symptoms of depression for more than two weeks, call your doctor:

- Feeling restless or moody

- Feeling sad, hopeless, and overwhelmed

- Crying a lot

- Having no energy or motivation

About This Chapter: Information in this chapter is from "Depression During and After Pregnancy," a publication of the Office on Women's Health, U.S. Department of Health and Human Services, March 2009.

- Eating too little or too much

- Sleeping too little or too much

- Having trouble focusing or making decisions

- Having memory problems

- Feeling worthless and guilty

- Losing interest or pleasure in activities you used to enjoy

- Withdrawing from friends and family

- Having headaches, aches and pains, or stomach problems that don't go away

It's A Fact!

Your doctor can figure out if your symptoms are caused by depression or something else.

What causes depression? What about postpartum depression?

There is no single cause. Rather, depression likely results from a combination of factors:

- Depression is a mental illness that tends to run in families. Women with a family history of depression are more likely to have depression.

- Changes in brain chemistry or structure are believed to play a big role in depression.

- Stressful life events, such as the death of a loved one, caring for an aging family member, abuse, and poverty can trigger depression.

- Hormonal factors unique to women may contribute to depression in some women. We know that hormones directly affect the brain chemistry that controls emotions and mood. We also know that women are at greater risk of depression at certain times in their lives, such as puberty, during and after pregnancy, and during perimenopause. Some women also have depressive symptoms right before their period.

Depression after childbirth is called postpartum depression. Hormonal changes may trigger symptoms of postpartum depression. When you are pregnant, levels of the female hormones estrogen and progesterone increase greatly. In the first 24 hours after childbirth, hormone levels quickly return to normal. Researchers think the big change in hormone levels may lead to depression. This is much like the way smaller hormone changes can affect a woman's moods before she gets her period.

Levels of thyroid hormones may also drop after giving birth. The thyroid is a small gland in the neck that helps regulate how your body uses and stores energy from food. Low levels of thyroid hormones can cause symptoms of depression. A simple blood test can tell if this condition is causing your symptoms. If so, your doctor can prescribe thyroid medicine.

Other factors may play a role in postpartum depression. You may feel the following:

- Tired after delivery
- Tired from a lack of sleep or broken sleep
- Overwhelmed with a new baby
- Doubts about your ability to be a good mother
- Stress from changes in work and home routines
- An unrealistic need to be a perfect mom
- Loss of who you were before having the baby
- Less attractive
- A lack of free time

Are some women more at risk for depression during and after pregnancy?

Certain factors may increase your risk of depression during and after pregnancy:

- A personal history of depression or another mental illness
- A family history of depression or another mental illness
- A lack of support from family and friends
- Anxiety or negative feelings about the pregnancy
- Problems with a previous pregnancy or birth
- Marriage or money problems
- Stressful life events
- Young age
- Substance abuse

Women who are depressed during pregnancy have a greater risk of depression after giving birth.

What is the difference between baby blues, postpartum depression, and postpartum psychosis?

Many women have the baby blues in the days after childbirth. If you have the baby blues, you may have the following symptoms:

- Mood swings
- Feeling sad, anxious, or overwhelmed
- Crying spells
- Loss of appetite
- Trouble sleeping

The baby blues most often go away within a few days or a week. The symptoms are not severe and do not need treatment.

> **Quick Tip**
>
> If you take medicine for depression, stopping your medicine when you become pregnant can cause your depression to come back. Do not stop any prescribed medicines without first talking to your doctor. Not using medicine that you need may be harmful to you or your baby.

The symptoms of postpartum depression last longer and are more severe. Postpartum depression can begin anytime within the first year after childbirth. If you have postpartum depression, you may have any of the symptoms of depression listed above. Symptoms may also include the following:

- Thoughts of hurting the baby
- Thoughts of hurting yourself
- Not having any interest in the baby

> **It's A Fact!**
>
> Postpartum depression needs to be treated by a doctor.

Postpartum psychosis is rare. It occurs in about one to four out of every 1,000 births. It usually begins in the first two weeks after childbirth. Women who have bipolar disorder or another mental health problem called schizoaffective disorder have a higher risk for postpartum psychosis. Symptoms may include the following:

- Seeing things that aren't there
- Feeling confused
- Having rapid mood swings

- Trying to hurt yourself or your baby

What should I do if I have symptoms of depression during or after pregnancy?

Call your doctor if any of the following are true:

- Your baby blues don't go away after two weeks
- Symptoms of depression get more and more intense
- Symptoms of depression begin any time after delivery, even many months later
- It is hard for you to perform tasks at work or at home
- You cannot care for yourself or your baby
- You have thoughts of harming yourself or your baby

Your doctor can ask you questions to test for depression. Your doctor can also refer you to a mental health professional who specializes in treating depression.

Some women don't tell anyone about their symptoms. They feel embarrassed, ashamed, or guilty about feeling depressed when they are supposed to be happy. They worry they will be viewed as unfit parents.

Any woman may become depressed during pregnancy or after having a baby. It doesn't mean you are a bad or not together mom. You and your baby don't have to suffer. There is help.

Here are some other helpful tips:

- Rest as much as you can. Sleep when the baby is sleeping.
- Don't try to do too much or try to be perfect.
- Ask your partner, family, and friends for help.
- Make time to go out, visit friends, or spend time alone with your partner.
- Discuss your feelings with your partner, family, and friends.
- Talk with other mothers so you can learn from their experiences.
- Join a support group. Ask your doctor about groups in your area.
- Don't make any major life changes during pregnancy or right after giving birth. Major changes can cause unneeded stress. Sometimes big changes can't be avoided. When that happens, try to arrange support and help in your new situation ahead of time.

How is depression treated?

There are two common types of treatment for depression:

- **Talk Therapy:** This involves talking to a therapist, psychologist, or social worker to learn to change how depression makes you think, feel, and act.

- **Medicine:** Your doctor can prescribe an antidepressant medicine. These medicines can help relieve symptoms of depression.

These treatment methods can be used alone or together. If you are depressed, your depression can affect your baby. Getting treatment is important for you and your baby. Talk with your doctor about the benefits and risks of taking medicine to treat depression when you are pregnant or breastfeeding.

What can happen if depression is not treated?

Untreated depression can hurt you and your baby. Some women with depression have a hard time caring for themselves during pregnancy. They may do the following:

- Eat poorly

- Not gain enough weight

- Have trouble sleeping

- Miss prenatal visits

- Not follow medical instructions

- Use harmful substances, like tobacco, alcohol, or illegal drugs

Depression during pregnancy can raise the risk of the following:

- Problems during pregnancy or delivery

- Having a low birthweight baby

- Premature birth

Untreated postpartum depression can affect your ability to parent. You may have the following problems:

- Lack of energy

- Trouble focusing

- Feeling moody

- Being unable to meet your child's needs

As a result, you may feel guilty and lose confidence in yourself as a mother. These feelings can make your depression worse.

Researchers believe postpartum depression in a mother can affect her baby. It can cause the baby to have the following problems:

- Delays in language development

- Problems with mother-child bonding

- Behavior problems

- Increased crying

It helps if your partner or another caregiver can help meet the baby's needs while you are depressed.

All children deserve the chance to have a healthy mom. And all moms deserve the chance to enjoy their life and their children. If you are feeling depressed during pregnancy or after having a baby, don't suffer alone. Please tell a loved one and call your doctor right away.

Chapter 22

Medicines And Pregnancy

Is it safe to use medicine while I am pregnant?

There is no clear-cut answer to this question. Before you start or stop any medicine, it is always best to speak with the doctor who is caring for you while you are pregnant. Read on to learn about deciding to use medicine while pregnant.

How should I decide whether to use a medicine while I am pregnant?

When deciding whether or not to use a medicine in pregnancy, you and your doctor need to talk about the medicine's benefits and risks.

- **Benefits:** What are the good things the medicine can do for me and my growing baby (fetus)?

- **Risks:** What are the ways the medicine might harm me or my growing baby (fetus)?

There may be times during pregnancy when using medicine is a choice. Some of the medicine choices you and your doctor make while you are pregnant may differ from the choices you make when you are not pregnant. For example, if you get a cold, you may decide to live with your stuffy nose instead of using the stuffy nose medicine you use when you are not pregnant.

Other times, using medicine is not a choice—it is needed. Some women need to use medicines while they are pregnant. Sometimes, women need medicine for a few days or a couple of weeks to treat a problem like a bladder infection or strep throat. Other women

---

About This Chapter: Information in this chapter is from "Pregnancy and Medicines," a publication of the Office on Women's Health, U.S. Department of Health and Human Services, April 2010.

need to use medicine every day to control long-term health problems like asthma, diabetes, depression, or seizures. Also, some women have a pregnancy problem that needs treatment with medicine. These problems might include severe nausea and vomiting, earlier pregnancy losses, or preterm labor.

Where do doctors and nurses find out about using medicines during pregnancy?

Doctors and nurses get information from medicine labels and packages, textbooks, and research journals. They also share knowledge with other doctors and nurses and talk to the people who make and sell medicines.

The Food and Drug Administration (FDA) is the part of our country's government that controls the medicines that can and can't be sold in the United States. The FDA lets a company sell a medicine in the United States if it is safe to use and works for a certain health problem. Companies that make medicines usually have to show FDA doctors and scientists whether birth defects or other problems occur in baby animals when the medicine is given to pregnant animals. Most of the time, drugs are not studied in pregnant women.

The FDA works with the drug companies to make clear and complete medicine labels. But in most cases, there is not much information about how a medicine affects pregnant women and their growing babies. Many prescription medicine labels include the results of studies done in pregnant animals. But a medicine does not always affect growing humans and animals in the same way.

How do prescription and over-the-counter (OTC) medicine labels help my doctor choose the right medicine for me when I am pregnant?

Doctors use information from many sources when they choose medicine for a patient, including medicine labels. To help doctors, the FDA created pregnancy letter categories to help explain what is known about using medicine during pregnancy. This system assigns letter categories to all prescription medicines. The letter category is listed on the label of a prescription medicine. The label states whether studies were done in pregnant women or pregnant animals and if so, what happened. Over-the-counter (OTC) medicines do not have a pregnancy letter category. Some OTC medicines were prescription medicines first and used to have a letter category. Talk to your doctor and follow the instructions on the label before taking OTC medicines.

The FDA is working hard to gather more knowledge about using medicine during pregnancy. The FDA is also trying to make medicine labels more helpful to doctors. Medicine label information for prescription medicines is now changing, and the pregnancy part of the label will change over the next few years. As this prescription information is updated, it is added to an online information clearinghouse called DailyMed (http://dailymed.nlm.nih.gov) that gives up-to-date, free information to consumers and health care providers.

It's A Fact!

Keep in mind that things like caffeine, vitamins, and herbal remedies can affect the growing fetus. Talk with your doctor about cutting down on caffeine and ask which type of vitamin you should take. Never use an herbal product without talking to your doctor first.

OTC Medicines: All OTC medicines have a Drug Facts label. The Drug Facts label is arranged the same way on all OTC medicines. This makes information about using the medicine easier to find. One section of the Drug Facts label is for pregnant women. With OTC medicines, the label usually tells a pregnant woman to speak with her doctor before using the medicine. Some OTC medicines are known to cause certain problems in pregnancy. The labels for these medicines give pregnant women facts about why and when they should not use the medicine. Here are some examples:

- Nonsteroidal anti-inflammatory drugs (NSAIDs) like ibuprofen (Advil, Motrin), naproxen (Aleve), and aspirin (acetylsalicylate), can cause serious blood flow problems in the baby if used during the last three months of pregnancy (after 28 weeks). Also, aspirin may increase the chance for bleeding problems in the mother and the baby during pregnancy or at delivery.

- The labels for nicotine therapy drugs, like the nicotine patch and lozenge, remind women that smoking can harm an unborn child. While the medicine is thought to be safer than smoking, the risks of the medicine are not fully known. Pregnant smokers are told to try quitting without the medicine first.

What if I get sick and need to use medicine while I am pregnant?

Whether or not you should use medicine during pregnancy is a serious question to discuss with your doctor. Some health problems need treatment. Not using a medicine that you need could harm you and your baby. For example, a urinary tract infection (UTI) that is not treated may become a kidney infection. Kidney infections can cause preterm labor and low birth-weight. You need an antibiotic to cure a UTI. Ask your doctor whether the benefits of taking a certain medicine outweigh the risks for you and your baby.

I have a health problem. Should I stop using my medicine while I am pregnant?

If you are pregnant or thinking about becoming pregnant, you should talk to your doctor about your medicines. Do not stop or change them on your own. This includes medicines for depression, asthma, diabetes, seizures (epilepsy), and other health problems. Not using medicine that you need may be more harmful to you and your baby than using the medicine.

If a diabetic woman does not use her medicine during pregnancy, she raises her risk for miscarriage, stillbirth, and some birth defects. If asthma and high blood pressure are not controlled during pregnancy, problems with the fetus may result.

It's A Fact!

For women living with human immunodeficiency virus (HIV), the Centers for Disease Control and Prevention (CDC) recommends using zidovudine (AZT) during pregnancy. Studies show that HIV positive women who use AZT during pregnancy greatly lower the risk of passing HIV to their babies.

Are vitamins safe for me while I am pregnant?

Women who are pregnant should not take regular vitamins. They can contain doses that are too high. Ask about special vitamins for pregnant women that can help keep you and your baby healthy. These prenatal vitamins should contain at least 400–800 micrograms of folic acid. It is best to start taking these vitamins before you become pregnant or if you could become pregnant. Folic acid reduces the chance of a baby having a neural tube defect, like spina bifida, where the spine or brain does not form the right way. Iron can help prevent a low red blood cell count (anemia). It's important to take the vitamin dose prescribed by your doctor. Too many vitamins can harm your baby. For example, very high levels of vitamin A have been linked with severe birth defects.

Are herbs, minerals, or amino acids safe for me while I am pregnant?

No one is sure if these are safe for pregnant women, so it's best not to use them. Even some natural products may not be good for women who are pregnant or breastfeeding. Except for

An Ounce Of Prevention: Vaccines And Pregnancy

Vaccines protect your body against dangerous diseases. Some vaccines are not safe to receive during pregnancy. For some vaccines, the decision to use it during pregnancy depends on the woman's own situation. Her doctor may consider these questions before giving a vaccine:

- Is there a high chance she will be exposed to the disease?
- Would the infection pose a risk to the mother or fetus?
- Is the vaccine unlikely to cause harm?

Talk with your doctor to make sure you are fully protected. The Centers for Disease Control and Prevention (CDC) provides vaccine guidelines for pregnant women.

some vitamins, little is known about using dietary supplements while pregnant. Some herbal remedy labels claim that they will help with pregnancy. But, most often there are no good studies to show if these claims are true or if the herb can cause harm to you or your baby. Talk with your doctor before using any herbal product or dietary supplement. These products may contain things that could harm you or your growing baby during your pregnancy.

In the United States, there are different laws for medicines and for dietary supplements. The part of the FDA that controls dietary supplements is the same part that controls foods sold in the United States. Only dietary supplements containing new dietary ingredients that were not marketed before October 15, 1994 submit safety information for review by the FDA. However, unlike medicines, the FDA does not approve herbal remedies and natural products for safety or for what they say they will do. Most have not even been evaluated for their potential to cause harm to you or the growing fetus, let alone shown to be safe for use in pregnancy. Before a company can sell a medicine, the company must complete many studies and send the results to the FDA. Many scientists and doctors at the FDA check the study results. The FDA allows the medicine to be sold only if the studies show that the medicine works and is safe to use.

Quick Tip

If you are pregnant and are using a medicine or were using one when you got pregnant, check to see if there is a pregnancy exposure registry for that medicine. The Food and Drug Administration has a list of pregnancy exposure registries at http://www.fda.gov/ScienceResearch/SpecialTopics/WomensHealthResearch/ucm134848.htm that pregnant women can join.

Chapter 23

X-Rays During Pregnancy

Pregnancy is a time to take good care of yourself and your unborn child. Many things are especially important during pregnancy, such as eating right, cutting out cigarettes and alcohol, and being careful about the prescription and over-the-counter drugs you take. Diagnostic x-rays and other medical radiation procedures of the abdominal area also deserve extra attention during pregnancy. This chapter is to help you understand the issues concerning x-ray exposure during pregnancy.

Diagnostic x-rays can give the doctor important and even life-saving information about a person's medical condition. But like many things, diagnostic x-rays have risks as well as benefits. They should be used only when they will give the doctor information needed to treat you.

You'll probably never need an abdominal x-ray during pregnancy. But sometimes, because of a particular medical condition, your physician may feel that a diagnostic x-ray of your abdomen or lower torso is needed. If this should happen, don't be upset. The risk to you and your unborn child is very small, and the benefit of finding out about your medical condition is far greater. In fact, the risk of not having a needed x-ray could be much greater than the risk from the radiation. But even small risks should not be taken if they're unnecessary.

You can reduce those risks by telling your doctor if you are, or think you might be, pregnant whenever an abdominal x-ray is prescribed. If you are pregnant, the doctor may decide that it would be best to cancel the x-ray examination, to postpone it, or to modify it to reduce the amount of radiation. Or, depending on your medical needs, and realizing that the risk is very small, the doctor may feel that it is best to proceed with the x-ray as planned. In any case, you should feel free to discuss the decision with your doctor.

About This Chapter: Information in this chapter is from "X-Rays, Pregnancy and You," a publication of the Food and Drug Administration, HHS Publication No. (FDA) 94-8087, March 2010.

X-Rays That Can Affect The Unborn Child

During most x-ray examinations—like those of the arms, legs, head, teeth, or chest—your reproductive organs are not exposed to the direct x-ray beam. So these kinds of procedures, when properly done, do not involve any risk to the unborn child. However, x-rays of the mother's lower torso—abdomen, stomach, pelvis, lower back, or kidneys—may expose the unborn child to the direct x-ray beam. They are of more concern.

The Possible Effects Of X-Rays

There is scientific disagreement about whether the small amounts of radiation used in diagnostic radiology can actually harm the unborn child, but it is known that the unborn child is very sensitive to the effects of things like radiation, certain drugs, excess alcohol, and infection. This is true, in part, because the cells are rapidly dividing and growing into specialized cells and tissues. If radiation or other agents were to cause changes in these cells, there could be a slightly increased chance of birth defects or certain illnesses, such as leukemia, later in life.

If you are x-rayed before you know you're pregnant, don't be alarmed. Remember that the possibility of any harm to you and your unborn child from an x-ray is very small. There are, however, rare situations in which a woman who is unaware of her pregnancy may receive a very large number of abdominal x-rays over a short period. Or she may receive radiation treatment of the lower torso. Under these circumstances, the woman should discuss the possible risks with her doctor.

How You Can Help Minimize The Risks

Most important, tell your physician if you are pregnant or think you might be. This is important for many medical decisions, such as drug prescriptions and nuclear medicine procedures, as well as x-rays. And remember, this is true even in the very early weeks of pregnancy.

Occasionally, a woman may mistake the symptoms of pregnancy for the symptoms of a disease. If you have any of the symptoms of pregnancy—nausea, vomiting, breast tenderness, fatigue—consider whether you might be pregnant and tell your doctor or x-ray technologist

It's A Fact!
The majority of birth defects and childhood diseases occur even if the mother is not exposed to any known harmful agent during pregnancy. Scientists believe that heredity and random errors in the developmental process are responsible for most of these problems.

(the person doing the examination) before having an x-ray of the lower torso. A pregnancy test may be called for.

If you are pregnant, or think you might be, do not hold a child who is being x-rayed. If you are not pregnant and you are asked to hold a child during an x-ray, be sure to ask for a lead apron to protect your reproductive organs. This is to prevent damage to your genes that could be passed on and cause harmful effects in your future descendants.

Whenever an x-ray is requested, tell your doctor about any similar x-rays you have had recently. It may not be necessary to do another. It is a good idea to keep a record of the x-ray examinations you and your family have had taken so you can provide this kind of information accurately.

Quick Tip

Feel free to talk with your doctor about the need for an x-ray examination. You should understand the reason x-rays are requested in your particular case.

Chapter 24

Drinking Alcohol During Pregnancy

Drinking alcohol during pregnancy can cause a wide range of physical and mental birth defects. The term "fetal alcohol spectrum disorders" (FASDs) is used to describe the many problems associated with exposure to alcohol before birth. Each year in the United States, up to 40,000 babies are born with FASDs.

Although many women are aware that heavy drinking during pregnancy can cause birth defects, many do not realize that moderate or even light drinking also may harm the fetus. In fact, no level of alcohol use during pregnancy has been proven safe. Therefore, the March of Dimes recommends that pregnant women do not drink any alcohol, including beer, wine, wine coolers, and liquor, throughout their pregnancy and while nursing. In addition, because women often do not know they are pregnant for a few months, women who may be pregnant or those who are attempting to become pregnant should not drink alcohol.

Recent government surveys indicate that about one in 12 pregnant women drink during pregnancy. About one in 30 pregnant women report binge drinking (five or more drinks on any one occasion). Women who binge drink or drink heavily greatly increase the risk of alcohol-related damage to their babies.

When a pregnant woman drinks, alcohol passes through the placenta to her fetus. In the fetus's immature body, alcohol is broken down much more slowly than in an adult's body. As a result, the alcohol level of the baby's blood can be higher and remain elevated longer than the level in the mother's blood. This sometimes causes the baby to suffer lifelong damage.

About This Chapter: Information in this chapter is from "Drinking Alcohol During Pregnancy," © 2008 March of Dimes Birth Defects Foundation. All rights reserved. For additional information, contact the March of Dimes at their website www.marchofdimes.com.

What are the hazards of drinking alcohol during pregnancy?

Drinking alcohol during pregnancy can cause FASDs, with effects that range from mild to severe. These effects include mental retardation; learning, emotional, and behavioral problems; and defects involving the heart, face, and other organs. The most severe of these effects is fetal alcohol syndrome (FAS), a combination of physical and mental birth defects.

Drinking alcohol during pregnancy increases the risk for miscarriage and premature birth (before 37 completed weeks of pregnancy). Studies also suggest that drinking during pregnancy may contribute to stillbirth. A 2008 Danish study found that women who binge drink three or more times during the first 16 weeks of pregnancy had a 56 percent greater risk for stillbirth than women who did not binge drink. Another 2008 study found that women who had five or more drinks a week were 70 percent more likely to have a stillborn baby than non-drinking women.

What is fetal alcohol syndrome (FAS)?

FAS is one of the most common known causes of mental retardation. It is the only cause that is entirely preventable. Studies by the Centers for Disease Control and Prevention (CDC) suggest that between 1,000 and 6,000 babies in the United States are born yearly with FAS.

Babies with FAS are abnormally small at birth and usually do not catch up on growth as they get older. They have characteristic facial features, including small eyes, a thin upper lip, and smooth skin in place of the normal groove between the nose and upper lip. Their organs, especially the heart, may not form properly. Many babies with FAS also have a brain that is small and abnormally formed. Most have some degree of mental disability. Many have poor coordination, a short attention span, and emotional and behavioral problems.

The effects of FAS and other FASDs last a lifetime. Even if not mentally retarded, adolescents and adults with FAS and other FASDs are at risk for psychological and behavioral problems and criminal behavior. They often find it difficult to keep a job and live independently.

What are other FASDs?

The CDC estimates that about three times the number of babies born with FAS are born with some, but not all, of the features of FAS. These FASDs are referred to as alcohol-related birth defects (ARBDs) and alcohol-related neurodevelopmental disorders (ARNDs).

- The term ARBDs describes physical birth defects that can occur in many organ systems, including the heart, liver, kidneys, eyes, ears, and bones.

- The term ARNDs describes learning and behavioral problems associated with prenatal exposure to alcohol. These problems can include learning disabilities; difficulties with attention, memory, and problem solving; speech and language delays; hyperactivity; psychological disorders; and poor school performance.

Children with ARBDs and ARNDs do not have the characteristic facial features associated with FAS.

In general, ARBDs are more likely to result from drinking alcohol during the first trimester, when organs are forming rapidly. Drinking at any stage of pregnancy can affect the brain, resulting in ARNDs, and can also affect growth.

An older term called fetal alcohol effects (FAEs) is sometimes used to describe alcohol-related damage that is less severe than FAS. The more specific diagnostic categories of ARBDs and ARNDs are now more frequently used.

How much alcohol is too much during pregnancy?

No level of drinking alcohol has been proven safe during pregnancy. According to the U.S. Surgeon General, the patterns of drinking that place a baby at greatest risk for FASDs are binge drinking and drinking seven or more drinks per week. However, FASDs can occur in babies of women who drink less.

- A 2002 study found that 14-year-old children whose mothers drank as little as one drink a week were significantly shorter and leaner and had a smaller head circumference (a possible indicator of brain size) than children of women who did not drink at all.

- A 2001 study found that six- and seven-year-old children of mothers who had as little as one drink a week during pregnancy were more likely than children of non-drinkers to have behavior problems, such as aggressive and delinquent behaviors. These researchers found that children whose mothers drank any alcohol during pregnancy were more than three times as likely as unexposed children to demonstrate delinquent behaviors.

- A 2007 study suggested that female children of women who drank less than one drink a week were more likely to have behavioral and emotional problems at four and eight years of age. The study also suggested similar effects in boys, but at higher levels of drinking.

- Other studies report behavioral and learning problems in children exposed to moderate drinking during pregnancy, including attention and memory problems, hyperactivity, impulsivity, poor social and communication skills, psychiatric problems (including mood disorders), and alcohol and drug use.

> **It's A Fact!**
> Researchers are taking a closer look at the more subtle effects of moderate and light drinking during pregnancy.

Is there a cure for FASDs?

There is no cure for FASDs. However, a 2004 study found that early diagnosis (before six years of age) and being raised in a stable, nurturing environment can improve the long-term outlook for individuals with FASDs. Children who experienced these protective factors during their school years were two to four times more likely to avoid serious behavioral problems resulting in trouble with the law or confinement in a psychiatric institution.

If a pregnant woman has one or two drinks before she realizes she is pregnant, can it harm the baby?

It is unlikely that the occasional drink a woman takes before she realizes she is pregnant will harm her baby. The baby's brain and other organs begin developing around the third week of pregnancy, however, and are vulnerable to damage in these early weeks. Because no amount of alcohol has been proven safe during pregnancy, a woman should stop drinking immediately if she even suspects she could be pregnant, and she should not drink alcohol if she is trying to become pregnant.

Is it safe to drink alcohol while breastfeeding?

Small amounts of alcohol do get into breastmilk and are passed on to the baby. One study found that breastfed babies of women who had one or more drinks a day were a little slower in acquiring motor skills (such as crawling and walking) than babies who had not been exposed to alcohol. Large amounts of alcohol may interfere with ejection of milk from the breast.

> **It's A Fact!**
> Because there currently is no way to predict which babies will be damaged by alcohol, the safest course is not to drink alcohol at all during pregnancy and to avoid heavy drinking during childbearing years (because about 50 percent of pregnancies are unplanned). All women who are considering becoming pregnant should stop drinking alcohol. Heavy drinkers should avoid pregnancy until they believe they can abstain from alcohol throughout pregnancy.

For these reasons, the March of Dimes recommends that women not drink alcohol while they are breastfeeding. Similarly, the American Academy of Pediatrics (AAP) recommends that breastfeeding mothers not drink alcohol. However, according to the AAP, an occasional alcoholic drink probably doesn't hurt the baby, but a mother who has a drink should wait at least two hours before breastfeeding her baby.

Can heavy drinking by the father contribute to FASDs?

There is no proof that heavy drinking by the father can cause FASDs. But men can help their partner avoid alcohol by not drinking during their partner's pregnancy.

What is the March of Dimes doing to prevent and treat FASDs?

March of Dimes-supported researchers are investigating the influence of alcohol on pregnancy.

- One grantee is seeking to identify genes that may play a role in causing FAS in order to identify women who are at high risk of having an affected baby if they continue to drink. This could make it possible to provide counseling that may help prevent FAS in their offspring.

- Another is seeking to determine the mechanism by which alcohol causes birth defects. This could lead to treatments to reverse or prevent further alcohol-related damage in pregnant women who drank alcohol before they knew they were pregnant or those who do not stop drinking.

The March of Dimes also works to prevent FASDs by educating the general public, teenagers, adults of childbearing age, and expectant mothers about the dangers of alcohol and other drugs to their unborn children.

Where can a woman get help to stop drinking alcohol?

Some women find it difficult to stop drinking. These organizations can help:

- National Council on Alcoholism and Drug Dependence (NCADD), (800) NCA-CALL (622-2255)
- Substance Abuse Treatment Facility Locator, (800) 622-HELP (4357)

Chapter 25

Smoking During Pregnancy

Like drinking too much alcohol or doing drugs, smoking is also very harmful to your health. It can cause serious health conditions including cancer, heart disease, stroke, and gum disease. It can also cause eye diseases that can lead to blindness. Smoking can make it harder for a woman to get pregnant.

Smoking And Your Baby

Not only is smoking harmful to you, it's also harmful to your baby during pregnancy. When you smoke during pregnancy, your baby is exposed to dangerous chemicals like nicotine, carbon monoxide, and tar. These chemicals can lessen the amount of oxygen that your baby gets. Oxygen is very important for helping your baby grow healthy. Smoking can also damage your baby's lungs.

Women who smoke during pregnancy are more likely to have:

- An ectopic pregnancy

- Vaginal bleeding

- Placental abruption (placenta peels away, partially or almost completely, from the uterine wall before delivery)

- Placenta previa (a low-lying placenta that covers part or all of the opening of the uterus)

- A stillbirth

About This Chapter: Information in this chapter is from "Smoking during Pregnancy," © 2010 March of Dimes Birth Defects Foundation. All rights reserved. For additional information, contact the March of Dimes at their website www.marchofdimes.com.

Babies born to women who smoke during pregnancy are more likely to be born:

- With birth defects such as cleft lip or palate
- Prematurely
- At low birthweight
- Underweight for the number of weeks of pregnancy

Secondhand Smoke

Breathing in someone else's smoke is also harmful. Secondhand smoke during pregnancy can cause a baby to be born at low birthweight. Secondhand smoke is also dangerous to young children. Babies exposed to secondhand smoke:

- Are more likely to die from SIDS (sudden infant death syndrome)
- Are at greater risk for asthma, bronchitis, pneumonia, ear infections, respiratory symptoms
- May experience slow lung growth

Thirdhand Smoke

New research shows that thirdhand smoke is another health hazard. Thirdhand smoke is made up of the toxic gases and particles left behind from cigarette or cigar smoking. These toxic remains, which include lead, arsenic, and carbon monoxide, cling to things like clothes, hair, couches, and carpets well after the smoke from a cigarette or cigar has cleared the room. That's why you often can tell a smoker by the smell of cigarettes or cigars that linger on his clothing or in his home or car. Things like cracking the car window down while you smoke or smoking in another room aren't enough to keep others away from the harm caused by cigarettes or cigars.

Breathing in these toxins at an early age (babies and young children) may have devastating health problems like asthma and other breathing issues, learning disorders, and cancer. It's important that expecting moms and their children do their best to keep away from places where people smoke.

It's A Fact!

Babies born prematurely and at low birthweight are at risk of other serious health problems, including lifelong disabilities (such as cerebral palsy, mental retardation, and learning problems), and in some cases, death.

Reasons To Quit

The sooner you quit smoking during pregnancy, the healthier you and your baby will be. It's best to quit smoking before getting pregnant. But if you're pregnant, this would be a great opportunity to kick the habit.

Some women may mistakenly think that switching to light or mild cigarettes are a safer choice during pregnancy. Other pregnant women may want to cut down on smoking rather than quitting altogether. It's true that the less you smoke, the better off baby will be. But quitting smoking is the best way to help ensure a healthy pregnancy and healthy baby.

Besides, when you quit smoking, you'll never again have to go outside and look for a place to smoke. You'll also have:

- Cleaner teeth

- Fresher breath

- Fewer stain marks on your fingers

- Fewer skin wrinkles

- A better sense of smell and taste

- More strength and ability to be more active

Tips To Quit

- Write down your reasons for quitting. Look at the list when you are tempted to smoke.

- Choose a quit day. On that day, throw away all your cigarettes or cigars, lighters, and ashtrays.

- Drink plenty of water.

- Keep your hands busy using a small stress ball or doing some needlework.

- Keep yourself occupied, too. Try going for a walk or doing chores to keep your mind off of cravings.

- Snack on some raw veggies or chew some sugarless gum to ease the need to have something in your mouth.

- Stay away from places, activities, or people that make you feel like smoking.

- Ask your partner or a friend to help you quit. Call that person when you feel like smoking.

- Ask your health care provider about quitting aids such as patches, gum, nasal spray, and medications.

- Don't start using these without your health care provider's okay, especially if you're pregnant.

- Don't get discouraged if you don't quit completely right away. Keep trying. If you can't quit, cut back as much as you can.

- Ask your employer to see what services are offered or covered by insurance.

- Learn about smoking cessation programs in your community or from your employer. You can get more information from you health care provider, hospital, or health department.

Chapter 26

Caffeine Use During Pregnancy

Caffeine is one of the most loved stimulants in America. But now that you are pregnant, you may need to lighten up on the daily intake of your favorite drinks and treats.

Facts About Caffeine

Caffeine is a stimulant and a diuretic. Because caffeine is a stimulant, it increases your blood pressure and heart rate, both of which are not recommended during pregnancy. Caffeine also increases the frequency of urination. This causes reduction in your body fluid levels and can lead to dehydration.

Caffeine crosses the placenta to your baby. Although you may be able to handle the amounts of caffeine you feed your body, your baby cannot. Your baby's metabolism is still maturing and cannot fully metabolize the caffeine. Any amount of caffeine can also cause changes in your baby's sleep pattern or normal movement pattern in the later stages of pregnancy.

Caffeine is found in more than just coffee. Caffeine is not only found in coffee but also in tea, soda, chocolate, and even some over-the-counter medications that relieve headaches. Be aware of what you consume.

Fact Versus Myth

Statement: Caffeine causes birth defects in humans.

Facts: Numerous studies on animals have shown that caffeine can cause birth defects, pre-term delivery, reduced fertility, and increase the risk of low-birth weight offspring and other

About This Chapter: Information in this chapter is from "What's the Real Scoop on Caffeine During Pregnancy," © 2011 American Pregnancy Association (www.americanpregnancy.org). Reprinted with permission.

reproductive problems. There have not been any conclusive studies done on humans though. It is still better to play it safe when it comes to inconclusive studies.

Statement: Caffeine causes infertility.

Facts: Some studies have shown a link between high levels of caffeine consumption and delayed conception.

Statement: Caffeine causes miscarriages.

Facts: In 2008, two studies on the effects of caffeine related to miscarriage showed significantly different outcomes. In one study released by the *American Journal of Obstetrics and Gynecology*, it was found that women who consume 200 milligrams (mg) or more of caffeine daily are twice as likely to have a miscarriage as those who do not consume any caffeine.

In another study released by *Epidemiology*, there was no increased risk in women who drank a minimal amount of coffee daily (between 200–350 mg per day).

Due to conflicting conclusions from numerous studies, the March of Dimes states that until more conclusive studies are done, pregnant women should limit caffeine intake to less than 200 mg per day. This is equal to about one 12 ounce (oz) cup of coffee.

Statement: A pregnant woman should not consume ANY caffeine.

Facts: Experts have stated that moderate levels of caffeine have not been found to have a negative effect on pregnancy. The definition of moderate varies anywhere from 150 mg–300 mg a day.

The Amount Of Caffeine In Your Favorite Drinks And Snacks

- Starbucks Grande Coffee (16 oz) 400 mg
- Starbucks House Blend Coffee (16 oz) 259 mg
- Dr. Pepper (12 oz) 37 mg
- 7 Eleven Big Gulp Diet Coke (32 oz) 124 mg

Remember
Caffeine is a stimulant and can keep both you and your baby awake.

- 7 Eleven Big Gulp Coca-Cola (32 oz) 92 mg

- Ben & Jerry's Coffee Buzz Ice Cream (8 oz) 72 mg

- Baker's chocolate (1 oz) 26 mg

- Green tea (6 oz) 40 mg

- Black tea (6 oz) 45 mg

- Excedrin (per capsule) 65 mg

Too Much Caffeine

The less caffeine you consume, the better. Some experts say more than 150 mg of caffeine a day is too much, while others say more than 300 mg a day is too much. Avoiding caffeine as much as possible is your safest course of action. If you must get your fix, it is best to discuss this with your health care provider to make the healthiest choice for you and your baby.

Chapter 27

Illicit Drug Use During Pregnancy

Nearly four percent of pregnant women in the United States use illicit drugs such as marijuana, cocaine, Ecstasy and other amphetamines, and heroin. These and other illicit drugs may pose various risks for pregnant women and their babies. Some of these drugs can cause a baby to be born too small or too soon, or to have withdrawal symptoms, birth defects, or learning and behavioral problems.

Because many pregnant women who use illicit drugs also use alcohol and tobacco, which also pose risks to unborn babies, it often is difficult to determine which health problems are caused by a specific illicit drug. Additionally, illicit drugs may be prepared with impurities that may be harmful to a pregnancy.

Finally, pregnant women who use illicit drugs may engage in other unhealthy behaviors that place their pregnancy at risk, such as having extremely poor nutrition or developing sexually transmitted infections. All of these factors make it difficult to know exactly what the effects of illicit drugs are on pregnancy.

What are the risks with use of marijuana during pregnancy?

Marijuana is the most frequently used illicit drug among women of childbearing age in the United States. Some studies suggest that use of marijuana during pregnancy may slow fetal growth and slightly decrease the length of pregnancy (possibly increasing the risk of premature birth). These effects are seen mainly in women who use marijuana regularly (six or more times a week).

After delivery, some babies who were regularly exposed to marijuana before birth appear to undergo withdrawal-like symptoms, including excessive crying and trembling. These babies have difficulty with state regulation (the ability to easily adjust to touch and changes in their environment), are more sensitive to stimulation, and have poor sleep patterns.

Couples who are planning pregnancy should keep in mind that marijuana can reduce fertility in both men and women, making it more difficult to conceive.

What is the long-term outlook for babies exposed to marijuana before birth?

There have been a limited number of studies following marijuana-exposed babies through childhood. Some did not find any increased risk of learning or behavioral problems. However, others found that children who were exposed to marijuana before birth are more likely to have subtle problems that affect their ability to pay attention. Exposed children do not appear to have a decrease in IQ.

What are the risks with use of Ecstasy, methamphetamine, and other amphetamines during pregnancy?

The use of Ecstasy, methamphetamine, and other amphetamines has increased dramatically in recent years. There have been few studies on how Ecstasy may affect pregnancy. One small study did find a possible increase in congenital heart defects and, in females only, of a skeletal defect called clubfoot. Babies exposed to Ecstasy before birth also may face some of the same risks as babies exposed to other types of amphetamines.

Another commonly abused amphetamine is methamphetamine, also known as speed, ice, crank, and crystal meth. A 2006 study found that babies of women who used this drug were more than three times as likely than unexposed babies to grow poorly before birth. Even when born at term, affected babies tend to be born with low birthweight (less than 5 ½ pounds) and have a smaller-than-normal head circumference.

It's A Fact!

After delivery, some babies who were exposed to amphetamines before birth appear to undergo withdrawal-like symptoms, including jitteriness, drowsiness, and breathing problems.

Use of methamphetamine during pregnancy also increases the risk of pregnancy complications, such as premature birth and placental problems. There also have been cases of birth defects, including heart defects and cleft lip/palate, in exposed babies, but researchers do not yet know whether the drug contributed to these defects.

What is the long-term outlook for babies exposed to Ecstasy, methamphetamine, and other amphetamines before birth?

The long-term outlook for these children is not known. Children who are born with low birthweight are at increased risk of learning and other problems. Children with reduced head circumference are more likely to have learning problems than those with low birthweight and normal head size. More studies are needed to determine the long-term outlook for children exposed to amphetamines before birth.

What are the risks with use of heroin during pregnancy?

Women who use heroin during pregnancy greatly increase their risk of serious pregnancy complications. These risks include poor fetal growth, premature rupture of the membranes (the bag of waters that holds the fetus breaks too soon), premature birth, and stillbirth.

As many as half of all babies of heroin users are born with low birthweight. Many of these babies are premature and often suffer from serious health problems during the newborn period, including breathing problems. They also are at increased risk of lifelong disabilities.

Use of heroin in pregnancy may increase the risk of a variety of birth defects. What is not entirely clear is whether these effects are caused by the drug itself or related to the poor health behaviors that women who take heroin often have. The substances that the heroin often is mixed with when it is made also may play a role.

Most babies of heroin users show withdrawal symptoms during the three days after birth, including fever, sneezing, trembling, irritability, diarrhea, vomiting, continual crying, and seizures. These symptoms usually subside by one week of age. The severity of a baby's symptoms is related to how long the mother has been using heroin or other narcotics and how high a dose she has taken. The longer the baby's exposure in the womb and the greater the dose, the more severe the withdrawal. Babies exposed to heroin before birth also face an increased risk of sudden infant death syndrome (SIDS).

A pregnant woman who uses heroin should not attempt to suddenly stop taking the drug. This can put her baby at increased risk of death. She should consult a health care provider or drug-treatment center about treatment with a drug called methadone.

It's A Fact!

While heroin can be sniffed, snorted, or smoked, most users inject the drug into a muscle or vein. Pregnant women who share needles are at risk of contracting human immunodeficiency virus (HIV, the virus that causes acquired immune deficiency syndrome (AIDS)) and the hepatitis C virus. These infections can be passed on to the infant during pregnancy or at birth.

Infants born to mothers taking methadone have withdrawal symptoms that can be safely treated. Methadone-exposed babies have higher birthweights than babies born to women who continue to use heroin. It is important for families to be aware that infants who are withdrawing from narcotics, including methadone, may continue to have symptoms of withdrawal for weeks after discharge from the nursery. There are effective ways to reduce the baby's discomfort using pacifiers, swaddling, and cuddling. Parents and caregivers benefit from support from family and friends and should seek out assistance if they are feeling stressed or overwhelmed.

What is the long-term outlook for babies exposed to heroin before birth?

The outlook for these children depends on a number of factors, including whether they suffered serious prematurity-related or other complications. Some studies suggest that children exposed to heroin before birth are at increased risk of learning and behavioral problems.

What are the risks of use of "T's and Blues" and opioid painkillers during pregnancy?

This is the street name for a mixture of a prescription opioid (related to morphine) painkiller called pentazocine and an over-the-counter allergy medicine. Individuals who abuse the mixture inject it into a vein. Babies of women who use T's and Blues during pregnancy are at increased risk of slow growth and may suffer withdrawal symptoms.

Additional Information About Drugs And Pregnancy

Information about medications, herbal products, and other specific substances that may potentially harm a developing fetus is available from the Organization of Teratology Information Specialists (OTIS). Visit www.otispregnancy.org (under the Resources tab, click on OTIS Fact Sheets) or call 866-626-6847.

Babies of women who abuse prescription oral (taken by mouth) opioid painkillers, such as oxycodone (OxyContin), also may undergo withdrawal.

What are the risks with use of cocaine during pregnancy?

Cocaine use during pregnancy can affect a pregnant woman and her baby in many ways. During the early months of pregnancy, cocaine may increase the risk of miscarriage. Later in pregnancy, it may trigger preterm labor (labor that occurs before 37 completed weeks of pregnancy) or cause the baby to grow poorly. As a result, cocaine-exposed babies are more likely than unexposed babies to be born prematurely and with low birthweight. Premature and low-birthweight babies are at increased risk of health problems during the newborn period, lasting disabilities such as mental retardation and cerebral palsy, and even death. Cocaine-exposed babies also tend to have smaller heads, which generally reflect smaller brains and an increased risk of learning problems.

Some studies suggest that cocaine-exposed babies are at increased risk of birth defects involving the urinary tract and, possibly, other birth defects. Cocaine may cause an unborn baby to have a stroke, which can result in irreversible brain damage and sometimes death.

Cocaine use during pregnancy can cause placental problems, including placental abruption. In this condition, the placenta pulls away from the wall of the uterus before labor begins. This can lead to heavy bleeding that can be life threatening for both mother and baby. The baby may be deprived of oxygen and adequate blood flow when an abruption occurs. Prompt cesarean delivery, however, can prevent most deaths but may not prevent serious complications for the baby caused by lack of oxygen.

After birth, some babies who were regularly exposed to cocaine before birth may have mild behavioral disturbances. As newborns, some are jittery and irritable, and they may startle and cry at the gentlest touch or sound. These babies may be difficult to comfort and may be withdrawn or unresponsive. Other cocaine-exposed babies turn off surrounding stimuli by going into a deep sleep for most of the day. Generally, these behavioral disturbances are temporary and resolve over the first few months of life.

What is the long-term outlook for babies who were exposed to cocaine before birth?

Most children who were exposed to cocaine before birth have normal intelligence. This is encouraging, in light of earlier predictions that many of these children would be severely brain damaged. A 2004 study at Case Western Reserve University found that four-year-old children who were exposed to cocaine before birth scored just as well on intelligence tests as unexposed children.

> ## It's A Fact!
> Cocaine-exposed babies may be more likely than unexposed babies to die of SIDS. However, studies suggest that poor health practices that often accompany maternal cocaine use (such as use of other drugs and smoking) may play a major role in these deaths.

However, the Case Western and other studies suggest that cocaine may sometimes contribute to subtle learning and behavioral problems, including language delays and attention problems. A good home environment appears to help reduce these effects. A recent study also suggests that cocaine-exposed children grow at a slower rate through age 10 than unexposed children, suggesting some lasting effect on development.

What are the risks of "club drugs," such as phencyclidine (PCP, angel dust), ketamine (Special K) and lysergic acid diethylamide (LSD, acid)?

There are few studies on the risks of these drugs during pregnancy. Babies of mothers who used PCP in pregnancy may have withdrawal symptoms. Babies exposed before birth to PCP or ketamine may be at increased risk of learning and behavioral problems. There have been occasional reports of birth defects in babies of women who used LSD during pregnancy, but it is not known whether or not the drug contributed to the defects.

What are the risks of inhaling glues and solvents during pregnancy?

Individuals, pregnant or not, who inhale these substances risk liver, kidney, and brain damage and even death. Abusing these substances during pregnancy can contribute to miscarriage, slow fetal growth, preterm birth, and birth defects. They also may cause withdrawal symptoms in the newborn.

How can a woman protect her baby from the dangers of illicit drugs?

Birth defects and other problems caused by illicit drugs are completely preventable. The March of Dimes advises women who use illicit drugs to stop before they become pregnant or to delay pregnancy until they believe they can avoid the drug completely throughout pregnancy. The March of Dimes also encourages pregnant women who use illicit drugs (with the exception of heroin) to stop using the drug immediately, because of the harm continued drug use may cause. Women who use heroin should consult their health care provider or a drug treatment center about methadone treatment.

Where can someone find more information on stopping drug use?

To learn more, ask a health care provider or contact:

- National Council on Alcoholism and Drug Dependence: 800-622-2255

- Substance Abuse Treatment Facility Locator: 800-662-4357

Does the March of Dimes support research on illicit drug use during pregnancy?

The March of Dimes has supported a number of research grants on drug use during pregnancy. For example, a recent grantee was studying physical and behavioral reasons that motivate pregnant women to abuse drugs such as cocaine, in order to improve drug treatment programs for pregnant women and reduce the risks to their babies. The March of Dimes also produces a variety of information and educational materials that inform pregnant women and others of the dangers of using drugs during pregnancy.

Chapter 28

Environmental Risks And Pregnancy

There are more than 83,000 chemicals used in homes and businesses in this country, yet we have little information on how most of them may affect you and your baby during pregnancy. A small number of chemicals are harmful to your unborn baby. Most of these are found in the workplace, but certain pollutants that damage the air and water, as well as chemicals used at home, may pose a risk during pregnancy.

During pregnancy, you can inhale these chemicals, ingest them in food or drink, or, in some cases, absorb them through the skin. You have to come in contact with large amounts of dangerous chemicals for a long time in order for them to harm your baby.

Most workplaces take steps to limit worker contact with chemicals. However, we don't really know how most chemicals may affect your health. Talk to your health care provider about chemicals used in your workplace before pregnancy if possible. If you're thinking of getting pregnant, you may need extra protection at work or a change in your job duties to stay safe. This is especially important if you work in industries such as agriculture, manufacturing, dry cleaning, printing, pharmaceutical manufacturing, and health care. You also can take steps to protect yourself and your baby from pollutants and chemicals used at home.

What are the risks of lead exposure during pregnancy?

Lead is a metal that was used for many years in gasoline and house paint. Although lead still can be found in the environment, the amounts have decreased greatly since the 1970s

About This Chapter: Information in this chapter is from "Environmental risks and pregnancy," © 2010 March of Dimes Birth Defects Foundation. All rights reserved. For additional information, contact the March of Dimes at their website www.marchofdimes.com.

when the U.S. Environmental Protection Agency (EPA) banned its use in these products. Lead poses health risks for everyone, but young children and unborn babies are at greatest risk. If you come in contact with high levels of lead during pregnancy, your baby may be at risk for miscarriage, preterm birth, low birth weight, and developmental delays.

If you live in an older home, you may be exposed to lead in deteriorating lead-based paint. Many homes built before 1978 were painted with lead-based paint. As long as paint is not crumbling or peeling, it poses little risk. However, crumbling paint can make lead dust when the surface is touched, especially when it is sanded or scraped.

Quick Tip

If lead-based paint needs to be removed from your home, stay away until the removal is complete. Only experts should remove leaded paint. The EPA has information about lead and lead removal.

You also can be exposed to significant amounts of lead in drinking water if your home has lead pipes, lead solder on copper pipes, or brass faucets. Contact your local health department or water supplier to find out how to get pipes tested for lead. If you use well water, have your water tested regularly for lead and other contaminants. The EPA Safe Drinking Water Hotline at (800) 426-4791 has more information on home water testing.

The EPA recommends running water for 15 to 30 seconds before using it for drinking or cooking to help reduce lead levels. Water from the cold water pipe contains less lead than water from the hot pipe, so use cold water for drinking, cooking, and preparing baby formula. Many home filters don't remove lead, so look for a filter that is certified by http://www.nsf.org/ to remove lead.

Other possible sources of lead in the home include:

- Lead crystal glassware and some ceramic dishes. Don't use these items. Ceramics you buy in a store are generally safer than those made by craftspeople.

- Some arts and crafts supplies, including oil paints, ceramic glazes, and stained glass materials. Use lead-free acrylic or watercolor paints during pregnancy and breastfeeding.

- Vinyl miniblinds imported from other countries.

- Old painted toys and some new toys and jewelry. The U.S. Consumer Product Safety Commission has information on recalls.

- Cosmetics containing surma or kohl.

- Lead solder in cans of food imported from other countries.

- Some candies imported from Mexico.

- Certain folk remedies for upset stomach, including those containing greta and azarcon.

Many lipsticks contain traces of lead. A 2009 study by the U.S. Food and Drug Administration (FDA) found small amounts of lead in all brands of lipstick tested. The FDA doesn't consider these lead levels to be a safety concern and didn't release the names of any of the lipstick brands. The Campaign for Safe Cosmetics conducted a similar study in 2007. You can get more information from http://www.safecosmetics.org/.

If you work in a field that puts you in contact with large amounts of lead on the job (such as painters, plumbers, and those working in smelters, auto repair shops, battery manufacturing plants, or certain types of construction), change your clothing (including shoes) and shower at work to avoid bringing lead into the home. Wash contaminated clothing at work or wash it at home separately from the rest of your family's clothing.

Does mercury exposure pose a risk in pregnancy?

Mercury is a metal that is found in the environment. Elemental (pure) mercury and methylmercury are two forms of mercury that may pose risks in pregnancy.

Elemental mercury is used in thermometers, dental fillings, fluorescent light bulbs, and some batteries. Dental amalgam is a silver-colored material used to fill cavities in teeth. It contains elemental mercury, silver, and other metals. Amalgam fillings can release small amounts of mercury vapor that can be inhaled. The FDA considers amalgam safe in adults and children over age six. However, there are few studies on the safety of amalgam in pregnant women and their babies. Some countries (Norway, Sweden, and Denmark) recommend that dentists not use dental amalgam in pregnant women. If you're concerned about the use of amalgam, talk with your dentist.

If you work in a dental office or in an industry that uses mercury to make products (including electrical, chemical, and mining industries), talk with your health care provider and take all recommended precautions.

Methylmercury is formed when mercury in the air is deposited in water. The mercury comes from natural sources (such as volcanoes) and manmade sources (such as burning coal and other industrial pollution). Fish that swim in these waters often have methylmercury in their tissues. People come in contact with the mercury when they eat these fish. Eating fish is the main source of methylmercury exposure in humans.

Trace amounts of mercury are present in many types of fish, but it's mostly found in certain large fish. For this reason, the FDA and the EPA advise pregnant women not to eat swordfish, shark, king mackerel, and tilefish.

Limit the amount of albacore (white) tuna you eat to six ounces or less a week. All of these fish may contain enough mercury to harm your unborn baby's developing nervous system, sometimes leading to learning disabilities.

What other metals pose a risk in pregnancy?

Arsenic may be harmful to pregnancy. It enters the environment through natural sources (weathering of rock and forest fires) and manmade sources (mining and electronics manufacturing).

Although arsenic is a well-known poison, the small amounts normally found in the environment are unlikely to harm an unborn baby.

However, you may come in contact with higher levels of arsenic that may pose an increased risk of pregnancy problems, including miscarriage and birth defects. Long-term exposure in children may result in lowered IQ. You may be exposed to higher levels of arsenic if you:

- Work or live near metal smelters.

- Live in agricultural areas where arsenic fertilizers (now banned in the United States) were used on crops.

- Live near hazardous waste sites or incinerators.

- Drink well water containing high levels of arsenic (this can occur in the places described above and in other areas, including parts of New England and the Midwest, that have naturally high levels of arsenic in rock).

If you live in areas that may have high arsenic levels, you can protect yourself by:

- Limiting contact with soil.

- Getting well water tested for arsenic to check if it's safe to drink or drinking bottled water.

- Community water suppliers already test for arsenic. The EPA has more information about testing water for arsenic.

- Checking decks and outdoor playsets made before 2003. Before that time, arsenic was used in these products. The EPA recommends applying a penetrating stain or sealant to these items once every year or two to reduce your chances of coming in contact with arsenic.

- Changing out of work clothing and shoes exposed to arsenic before going home.

Can pesticides harm an unborn baby?

There is little proof that coming in contact with pest-control products (insecticides) at levels commonly used at home poses a risk to your unborn baby. However, all insecticides are to some extent poisonous. Some studies suggest that coming in contact with large amounts of pesticides may lead to miscarriage, preterm birth, low birth weight, birth defects, and learning problems. If you do agricultural work or live in agricultural areas, you may be more likely to come in contact with high levels of pesticides than other women. Avoid pesticides whenever possible.

What are solvents?

Solvents are chemicals that dissolve other substances. Solvents include alcohols, degreasers, paint thinners, and stain and varnish removers. Lacquers, silk-screening inks, and paints also contain these chemicals. A number of studies suggest that coming in contact with solvents at work may increase the risk of birth defects. A 1999 Canadian study found that women who were exposed to solvents on the job during their first trimester of pregnancy were 13 times more likely than unexposed women to have a baby with a major birth defect, like spina bifida (open spine), clubfoot, heart defects, and deafness. The women in the study included factory workers, laboratory technicians, artists, graphic designers, and printing industry workers.

Other studies have found that women workers in semiconductor plants exposed to high levels of solvents called glycol ethers were more likely than unexposed women to miscarry. Glycol ethers also are used in jobs that involve photography, dyes, and silkscreen printing.

If you work with solvents, even if you do arts and crafts at home, minimize your exposure by:

- Making sure your workplace is well ventilated

- Wearing appropriate protective clothing, including gloves and a face mask

- Avoiding meals or drinking in your work area

Quick Tip

To learn more about the chemicals you work with, ask your employer for their safety information sheets. These sheets, made by chemical manufacturers, include information about possible dangers of specific chemicals and recommended safety tips for people who work with them. The MSDSSearch has a list of these sheets. You also can visit the National Institute for Occupational Safety and Health.

Do household cleaning products pose a risk in pregnancy?

Although some household cleansers contain solvents, there are many safe alternatives. Read labels carefully and don't use products (such as some oven cleaners) whose labels state that they are toxic.

Products that contain ammonia or chlorine are unlikely to harm your unborn baby, although their odors may cause you nausea. Open windows and doors and wear rubber gloves when using these products. Never mix ammonia and chlorine products because the combination produces fumes that are dangerous for anyone.

If you're worried about household cleansers or bothered by their odors, you can use safe, natural products instead. For example, use baking soda as a powdered cleanser to scrub greasy areas, pots and pans, sinks, tubs, and ovens. You also can use a mixture of vinegar and water to clean many surfaces, such as countertops.

Do chemicals in plastics pose a risk to the fetus or infant?

Possibly. Plastics are made from a number of chemicals, including phthalates and bisphenol A (BPA). Phthalates make plastic soft and flexible. They are used in toys, medical devices (such as tubing), shampoos, cosmetics, and food packaging. BPA makes plastics clear and strong. It is used in baby bottles, food containers (to line metal food cans), and water bottles.

Recent research suggests that exposure to phthalates before birth may lead to subtle defects in male genitals. Phthalates also may pose a risk after birth. In 2006, the National Toxicology Program (NTP) concluded that one type of phthalate used in plastic medical tubing could pose a risk to the reproductive systems of baby boys. Many hospitals have removed such products from newborn nurseries. In 2008, the NTP also expressed concern about the effects of BPA on the brain, behavior, and prostate gland in fetuses, infants, and children. Other studies suggest that high BPA levels may play a role in some miscarriages.

Studies are continuing on possible health effects of these chemicals. Until there are better answers, you can take these steps to limit your exposure:

It's A Fact!

In 2009, the United States banned the use of some phthalates from toys and child care articles, including any product children age three and younger use for sleeping, feeding, sucking, or teething. Some manufacturers have discontinued use of BPA in baby bottles.

- Don't use plastic containers with the number seven or the letters PC (polycarbonate) in the triangle found on the bottom.

- Limit use of canned food.

- Don't microwave food in plastic containers or put plastics in the dishwasher.

You can limit your baby's exposure by:

- Breastfeeding your baby so you don't have to use baby bottles.

- Using baby bottles made of glass, polypropylene or polyethylene.

- Giving your baby plastic toys made after February 2009 or labeled phthalate-free.

- Limiting use of baby lotions or powders that contain phthalates.

Chapter 29

Abuse During Pregnancy

Abuse, whether emotional or physical, is never okay. Unfortunately, some women experience abuse from a partner. Abuse crosses all racial, ethnic, and economic lines. Abuse often gets worse during pregnancy. Almost one in six pregnant women have been abused by a partner.

What is abuse?

Abuse can come in many forms. An abusive partner may cause emotional pain by calling you names or constantly blaming you for something you haven't done. An abuser may try to control your behavior by not allowing you to see your family and friends, or by always telling you what you should be doing. Emotional abuse may lead you to feel scared or depressed, eat an unhealthy diet, or pick up bad habits such as smoking or drinking.

An abusive partner may try to hurt your body. This physical abuse can include hitting, slapping, kicking, choking, pushing, or even pulling your hair. Sometimes, an abuser will aim these blows at a pregnant woman's belly. This kind of violence not only can harm you, but it also can put your unborn baby in grave danger. During pregnancy, physical abuse can lead to miscarriage and vaginal bleeding. It can cause your baby to be born too soon, have low birthweight, or physical injuries.

What can trigger abuse during pregnancy?

For many families, pregnancy can bring about feelings of stress, which is normal. But it's not okay for your partner to react violently to stress. Some partners become abusive during pregnancy because they feel:

About This Chapter: Information in this chapter is from "Abuse during pregnancy," © 2008 March of Dimes Birth Defects Foundation. All rights reserved. For additional information, contact the March of Dimes at their website www.marchofdimes.com.

- Upset because this was an unplanned pregnancy

- Stressed at the thought of financially supporting a first baby or another baby

- Jealous that your attention may shift from your partner to your new baby, or to a new relationship

How do you know if you're in an abusive relationship?

It's common for couples to argue now and then. But violence and emotional abuse are different from the minor conflicts that couples have.

Ask yourself:

- Does my partner always put me down and make me feel bad about myself?

- Has my partner caused harm or pain to my body?

- Does my partner threaten me, the baby, my other children, or himself?

- Does my partner blame me for his actions? Does he tell me it's my own fault he hit me?

- Is my partner becoming more violent as time goes on?

- Has my partner promised never to hurt me again, but still does?

If you answered "Yes" to any of these questions, you may be in an unhealthy relationship.

What can you do?

Recognize that you are in an abusive relationship. Once you realize this, you've made the first step towards help. There are lots of things you can do.

Tell someone you trust. This can be a friend, a clergy member, a health care provider, or counselor. Once you've confided in them, they might be able to put you in touch with a crisis hotline, domestic violence program, legal-aid service, or a shelter or safe haven for abused women.

Have a plan for your safety. This can include:

- Learn the phone number of your local police department and health care provider's office in case your partner hurts you. Call 911 if you need immediate medical attention. Be sure to obtain a copy of the police or medical record should you choose to file charges against the abuser.

- Find a safe place. Talk to a trusted friend, neighbor, or family member that you can stay with, no matter what time of day or night, to ensure your safety.

Remember

No one deserves to be physically or emotionally abused. Recognize the signs of abuse and seek help. You might feel very scared at the thought of leaving, but you've got to do it. Your life and your baby's life depend on it.

- Put together some extra cash and any important documents or items you might need, such as a driver's license, health insurance cards, a checkbook, bank account information, Social Security cards, and prescription medications. Have these items in one safe place so you can take them with you quickly.

- Pack a suitcase with toiletries, an extra change of clothes for you and your children, and an extra set of house and car keys. Give the suitcase to someone you trust who can hold it for you safely.

For More Information

Learn more about domestic violence and abuse at Georgetown University's Maternal and Child Health Library.

If you need help, call the national domestic violence hotline: (800) 799-SAFE (7233), (800) 787-3224 TTY

Part Four
High-Risk Pregnancies And
Pregnancy Complications

Chapter 30

High-Risk Pregnancy

Risk Factors Present Before Pregnancy

Some risk factors are present before women become pregnant. These risk factors include certain physical and social characteristics of women, problems that have occurred in previous pregnancies, and certain disorders women already have.

Physical Characteristics

The following characteristics of women affect risk during pregnancy.

Age: Girls aged 15 and younger are at increased risk of preeclampsia (a type of high blood pressure that develops during pregnancy). Young girls are also at increased risk of preterm labor and anemia. They are more likely to have babies who have anemia or who are underweight (small for gestational age).

Women aged 35 and older are at increased risk of problems such as high blood pressure, gestational diabetes (diabetes that develops during pregnancy), chromosomal abnormalities in the fetus, and stillbirth. Also, they are more likely to have complications during labor such as preeclampsia, a placenta that detaches too soon (placental abruption) or is mislocated (placenta previa), and difficult labor.

Weight: Women who weigh less than 100 pounds before becoming pregnant are more likely to have small, underweight babies.

About This Chapter: This chapter includes "Risk Factors Present Before Pregnancy," and "Risk Factors That Develop During Pregnancy," from the *Merck Manual Home Health Handbook*, edited by Robert Porter. Copyright 2011 by Merck Sharp & Dohme Corp., a subsidiary of Merck & Co, Inc, Whitehouse Station, NJ. Available at http://www.merckmanuals.com/home/. Accessed August 2011.

Obese women are more likely to have very large babies, which may be difficult to deliver. Also, obese women are more likely to develop gestational diabetes, high blood pressure, or preeclampsia. They are more likely to have a pregnancy that lasts 42 weeks or longer (postterm) and to need a cesarean delivery.

Height: Women shorter than five feet are more likely to have a small pelvis, which may make movement of the fetus through the pelvis and vagina (birth canal) difficult during labor. For example, the fetus's shoulder is more likely to lodge against the pubic bone. This complication is called shoulder dystocia. Also, short women are more likely to have preterm labor and a baby who has not grown as much as expected.

Reproductive Abnormalities: Structural abnormalities in the uterus or cervix increase the risk of having a difficult labor, a miscarriage, or a fetus in an abnormal position and of needing a cesarean delivery. These abnormalities include a double uterus or a weak (incompetent) cervix that tends to open (dilate) as the fetus grows.

Social Characteristics

Being unmarried or in a lower socioeconomic group increases the risk of problems during pregnancy. The reason these characteristics increase risk is unclear but is probably related to other characteristics that are more common among these women. For example, these women are more likely to smoke and less likely to consume a healthy diet and to obtain appropriate medical care.

Problems In A Previous Pregnancy

When women have had a problem in one pregnancy, they are more likely to have a problem, often the same one, in subsequent pregnancies. Such problems include having had any of the following:

- A premature baby
- An underweight baby
- A baby that weighed more than 10 pounds
- A baby with birth defects
- A previous miscarriage
- A late (postterm) delivery (after 42 weeks of pregnancy)
- Rh incompatibility that required a blood transfusion to the fetus
- Labor that required a cesarean delivery

- A baby who died shortly before or after birth (stillbirth)

Women may have a condition that tends to make the same problem recur. For example, women with diabetes are more likely to have babies that weigh more than 10 pounds at birth.

Women who had a baby with a genetic disorder or birth defect are more likely to have another baby with a similar problem. Genetic testing of the baby, even if stillborn, and of both parents may be appropriate before another pregnancy is attempted. If these women become pregnant again, tests such as high-resolution ultrasonography, chorionic villus sampling, and amniocentesis may help determine whether the fetus has a genetic disorder or birth defect. These women may be referred to a specialist.

Having had five or more pregnancies increases the risk of very rapid labor and excessive bleeding after delivery. Having had twins or more fetuses in one pregnancy (multiple births) increases the risk of a mislocated placenta (placenta previa).

Disorders Present Before Pregnancy

Before becoming pregnant, women may have a disorder that can increase the risk of problems during pregnancy. These women should talk with a doctor and try to get in the best physical condition possible before they become pregnant. After they become pregnant, they may need special care, often from an interdisciplinary team. The team may include an obstetrician (who may also be a specialist in the disorder), a specialist in the disorder, and other health care practitioners (such as nutritionists).

Risk Factors That Develop During Pregnancy

During pregnancy, a problem may occur or a condition may develop to make the pregnancy high risk. For example, pregnant women may be exposed to something that can cause birth defects (teratogens), such as radiation, certain chemicals, drugs, or infections. Or a disorder may develop. Some disorders are related to (are complications of) pregnancy. Other disorders are not directly related to pregnancy. Certain disorders are more likely to occur during pregnancy because of the many changes pregnancy causes in a woman's body.

Drugs

Some drugs taken during pregnancy cause birth defects. Examples are isotretinoin (used to treat severe acne), some anticonvulsants, lithium, some antibiotics (such as streptomycin, kanamycin, and tetracycline), thalidomide, warfarin, and angiotensin-converting enzyme (ACE) inhibitors (if taken during the last two trimesters). Taking drugs that block the actions of folate (folic acid), such as the immunosuppressant methotrexate or the antibiotic trimethoprim, can also cause birth defects. A deficiency of folate increases the risk of having a baby with a birth defect. Early in pregnancy, women are asked if they are using any of these drugs.

Women are also asked if they use any recreational drugs. Of particular concern are alcohol, cocaine, and nicotine (in cigarette smoking). All of these drugs can cause miscarriage or cause the baby to be underweight or to have birth defects. These drugs have the following risks:

- **Alcohol:** The risk of mental retardation (intellectual disability) is increased. Fetal alcohol syndrome is also possible.

- **Cocaine:** The risk of premature detachment of the placenta (placental abruption), premature birth, and stillbirth is increased. The fetus may not grow as much as expected.

- **Smoking Cigarettes:** The risk of stillbirth and pregnancy complications, such as premature labor, placenta previa, placental abruption, and premature rupture of membranes, is increased. The fetus may not grow as much as expected, and children are more likely to have behavioral problems and mental retardation (intellectual disability).

Pregnancy Complications

Pregnancy complications are problems that occur only during pregnancy. They may affect the woman, the fetus, or both and may occur at different times during the pregnancy. For example, complications such as a mislocated placenta (placenta previa) or premature detachment of the placenta from the uterus (placental abruption) can cause bleeding from the vagina during pregnancy. Women who have heavy bleeding are at risk of losing the baby or of going into shock and, if not promptly treated, of dying during labor and delivery.

What can a woman do to promote a healthy pregnancy?

Many health care providers recommend that a woman who is thinking about becoming pregnant see a health care provider to ensure she is in good preconception health.

During pregnancy, there are also steps a woman can take to reduce the risk of certain problems:

- Getting at least 400 micrograms of folic acid every day if she thinks she could become pregnant, and continuing folic acid when she does get pregnant
- Getting proper immunizations
- Maintaining a healthy weight and diet, getting regular physical activity, and avoiding smoking, alcohol, or drug use
- Starting prenatal care appointments early in pregnancy

Source: From "High-Risk Pregnancy," a publication of the National Institute of Child Health and Human Development, 2006.

What are some conditions that may cause a high-risk pregnancy?

- **Preeclampsia And Eclampsia:** Preeclampsia is a syndrome that includes high blood pressure, urinary protein, and changes in blood levels of liver enzymes during pregnancy. It can affect the mother's kidneys, liver, and brain. With treatment, many women will have healthy babies. If left untreated, the condition can be fatal for the mother and/or the baby and can lead to long-term health problems. Eclampsia is a more severe form of preeclampsia that can cause seizures and coma in the mother.

- **Gestational Diabetes Mellitus (Or Gestational Diabetes):** A type of diabetes that only pregnant women get. If a woman gets diabetes when she is pregnant, but never had it before, then she has gestational diabetes. Many women with gestational diabetes have healthy pregnancies and healthy babies because they follow a treatment plan from their health care provider.

- **Human Immunodeficiency Virus/Acquired Immune Deficiency Syndrome (HIV/AIDS):** Kills or damages cells of the body's immune system, progressively destroying the body's ability to fight infections and certain cancers. The term AIDS applies to the most advanced stages of HIV infection. Women can give HIV to their babies during pregnancy, while giving birth, or through breastfeeding. But, there are effective ways to prevent the spread of mother-to-infant transmission of HIV.

- **Preterm Labor:** Labor that begins before 37 weeks of pregnancy. Because the baby is not fully grown at this time, it may not be able to survive outside the womb. Health care providers will often take steps to try to stop labor if it occurs before this time. Although there is no way to know which women will experience preterm labor or birth, there are factors that place women at higher risk, such as certain infections, a shortened cervix, or previous preterm birth.

- **Other Medical Conditions:** High blood pressure, diabetes, or heart, breathing, or kidney problems can become more serious during a woman's pregnancy. Regular prenatal care can help ensure a healthier pregnancy for a woman and her baby.

Source: From "High-Risk Pregnancy," a publication of the National Institute of Child Health and Human Development, 2006.

Chapter 31

Genetic Testing

Genetic tests are done by analyzing small samples of blood or body tissues. They determine whether you, your partner, or your baby carry genes for certain inherited disorders.

Genetic testing has developed enough so that doctors can often pinpoint missing or defective genes. The type of genetic test needed to make a specific diagnosis depends on the particular illness that a doctor suspects.

Many different types of body fluids and tissues can be used in genetic testing. For deoxyribonucleic acid (DNA) screening, only a very tiny bit of blood, skin, bone, or other tissue is needed.

Genetic Testing During Pregnancy

For genetic testing before birth, pregnant women may decide to undergo amniocentesis or chorionic villus sampling.

Amniocentesis is a test performed between weeks 16 and 18 of a woman's pregnancy. The doctor inserts a hollow needle into the woman's abdomen to remove a small amount of amniotic fluid from around the developing fetus. This fluid can be tested to check for genetic problems and to determine the sex of the child. When there's risk of cesarean section or premature birth, amniocentesis may also be done to see how far the child's lungs have matured. Amniocentesis carries a slight risk of inducing a miscarriage.

About This Chapter: Information in this chapter is from "Genetic Testing," June 2010, reprinted with permission from www.kidshealth.org. Copyright © 2010 The Nemours Foundation. This information was provided by KidsHealth, one of the largest resources online for medically reviewed health information written for parents, kids, and teens. For more articles like this one, visit www.KidsHealth.org, or www.TeensHealth.org.

Chorionic villus sampling (CVS) is usually performed between the 10th and 12th weeks of pregnancy. The doctor removes a small piece of the placenta to check for genetic problems in the fetus. Because chorionic villus sampling is an invasive test, there's a small risk that it can induce a miscarriage.

Why Doctors Recommend Genetic Testing

A doctor may recommend genetic counseling or testing for any of the following reasons:

- **A couple is planning to start a family and one of them or a close relative has an inherited illness.** Some people are carriers of genes for genetic illnesses, even though they don't show, or manifest, the illness themselves. This happens because some genetic illnesses are recessive—meaning that they're only expressed if a person inherits two copies of the problem gene, one from each parent. Offspring who inherit one problem gene from one parent but a normal gene from the other parent won't have symptoms of a recessive illness but will have a 50 percent chance of passing the problem gene on to their children.

- **An individual already has one child with a severe birth defect.** Not all children who have birth defects have genetic problems. Sometimes, birth defects are caused by exposure to a toxin (poison), infection, or physical trauma before birth. Even if a child does have a genetic problem, there's always a chance that it wasn't inherited and that it happened because of some spontaneous error in the child's cells, not the parents' cells.

- **A woman has had two or more miscarriages.** Severe chromosome problems in the fetus can sometimes lead to a spontaneous miscarriage. Several miscarriages may point to a genetic problem.

- **A woman has delivered a stillborn child with physical signs of a genetic illness.** Many serious genetic illnesses cause specific physical abnormalities that give an affected child a very distinctive appearance.

- **A woman is pregnant and over age 34.** Chances of having a child with a chromosomal problem (such as trisomy) increase when a pregnant woman is older. Older fathers are at risk to have children with new dominant genetic mutations (those that are caused by a single genetic defect that hasn't run in the family before).

- **A child has medical problems that might be genetic.** When a child has medical problems involving more than one body system, genetic testing may be recommended to identify the cause and make a diagnosis.

- **A child has medical problems that are recognized as a specific genetic syndrome.** Genetic testing is performed to confirm the diagnosis. In some cases, it also might aid in identifying the specific type or severity of a genetic illness, which can help identify the most appropriate treatment.

A Word Of Caution

Although advances in genetic testing have improved doctors' ability to diagnose and treat certain illnesses, there are still some limits. Genetic tests can identify a particular problem gene, but can't always predict how severely that gene will affect the person who carries it. In cystic fibrosis, for example, finding a problem gene on chromosome number 7 can't necessarily predict whether a child will have serious lung problems or milder respiratory symptoms.

Also, simply having problem genes is only half the story because many illnesses develop from a mix of high-risk genes and environmental factors. Knowing that you carry high-risk genes may actually be an advantage, if it gives you the chance to modify your lifestyle to avoid becoming sick.

As research continues, genes are being identified that put people at risk for illnesses like cancer, heart disease, psychiatric disorders, and many other medical problems. As research continues, the hope is that someday it will be possible to develop specific types of gene therapy to totally prevent some diseases and illnesses.

Gene therapy is already being used with limited success to treat cystic fibrosis and adenosine deaminase (ADA) deficiency (an immune deficiency). However, severe complications have occurred in some individuals receiving gene therapy, so current research with gene therapy is very carefully controlled and none involves children.

It's A Fact!

Sickle cell disease, thalassemias, and other blood disorders may be the next targets for a genetic cure. Although genetic treatments for major killers, like cancer, may be a long way off, there is still great hope that many more genetic cures will be found. The Human Genome Project, which was completed in 2003, identified and mapped out all of the genes (up to 25,000) carried in our human chromosomes. The map is just the start, but it's a very hopeful beginning.

Chapter 32

Pregnancy Complications

Complications of pregnancy are health problems that occur during pregnancy. They can involve the mother's health, the baby's health, or both. Some women have health problems before they become pregnant that could lead to complications. Other problems arise during the pregnancy. Keep in mind that whether a complication is common or rare, there are ways to manage problems that come up during pregnancy.

Health Problems Before Pregnancy

Before pregnancy, make sure to talk to your doctor about health problems you have now or have had in the past. If you are receiving treatment for a health problem, your doctor might want to change the way your health problem is managed. Some medicines used to treat health problems could be harmful if taken during pregnancy. At the same time, stopping medicines that you need could be more harmful than the risks posed should you become pregnant. Be assured that you are likely to have a normal, healthy baby when health problems are under control and you get good prenatal care.

Asthma

Poorly controlled asthma may increase risk of preeclampsia, poor weight gain in the fetus, preterm birth, cesarean birth, and other complications. If pregnant women stop using asthma medicine, even mild asthma can become severe.

About This Chapter: Information in this chapter is from "Pregnancy Complications," a publication of the Office on Women's Health, U.S. Department of Health and Human Services, September 2010.

Depression

Depression that persists during pregnancy can make it hard for a woman to care for herself and her unborn baby. Having depression before pregnancy also is a risk factor for postpartum depression.

Diabetes

High blood glucose (sugar) levels during pregnancy can harm the fetus and worsen a woman's long-term diabetes complications.

Epilepsy And Other Seizure Disorders

Seizures during pregnancy can harm the fetus, and increase the risk of miscarriage or stillbirth. But using medicine to control seizures might cause birth defects. For most pregnant women with epilepsy, using medicine poses less risk to their own health and the health of their babies than stopping medicine.

High Blood Pressure

Having chronic high blood pressure puts a pregnant woman and her baby at risk for problems. Women with high blood pressure have a higher risk of preeclampsia and placental abruption (when the placenta separates from the wall of the uterus). The likelihood of preterm birth and low birthweight also is higher.

Migraine

Migraine symptoms tend to improve during pregnancy. Some women have no migraine attacks during pregnancy. Certain medicines commonly used to treat headaches should not be used during pregnancy. A woman who has severe headaches should speak to her doctor about ways to relieve symptoms safely.

Overweight And Obesity

Recent studies suggest that the heavier a woman is before she becomes pregnant, the greater her risk of a range of pregnancy complications, including preeclampsia and preterm delivery. Overweight and obese women who lose weight before pregnancy are likely to have healthier pregnancies.

Thyroid Disease

Uncontrolled hyperthyroidism (overactive thyroid) can be dangerous to the mother and cause health problems such as heart failure and poor weight gain in the fetus. Uncontrolled hypothyroidism (underactive thyroid) also threatens the mother's health and can cause birth defects.

Pregnancy-Related Problems

Sometimes pregnancy problems arise—even in healthy women. Some prenatal tests done during pregnancy can help prevent these problems or spot them early. Call your doctor if you have any of the symptoms listed here. If a problem is found, make sure to follow your doctor's advice about treatment. Doing so will boost your chances of having a safe delivery and a strong, healthy baby.

Anemia

Anemia occurs when a person has a lower than normal number of healthy red blood cells. Symptoms include: feeling tired, faint, or weak; looking pale; and shortness of breath. Women with pregnancy-related anemia are helped by taking iron and folic acid supplements. Your doctor will check your iron levels throughout pregnancy to be sure anemia does not happen again.

Depression

Pregnancy-related depression is extreme sadness during pregnancy or after birth (postpartum). Symptoms include: intense sadness; helplessness and irritability; appetite changes; and thoughts of harming self or baby. Women who are pregnant might be helped with one or a combination of treatment options.

Gestational Diabetes

A woman with gestational diabetes has blood sugar levels that are too high during pregnancy. Usually, there are no symptoms. Sometimes, symptoms include extreme thirst, hunger, or fatigue. A screening test shows high blood sugar levels. Most women with pregnancy related diabetes can control their blood sugar levels by following a healthy meal plan from their doctor.

Pregnancy-Related High Blood Pressure

Pregnancy-related high blood pressure is high blood pressure that starts after 20 weeks of pregnancy and goes away after birth; high blood pressure without other signs and symptoms of preeclampsia. The health of the mother and baby are closely watched to make sure high blood pressure is not preeclampsia.

It's A Fact!
A mother's depression can affect her baby's development, so getting treatment is important for both mother and baby.

Hyperemesis Gravidarum (HG)

HG is severe, persistent nausea and vomiting during pregnancy. Symptoms include nausea that does not go away; vomiting several times every day; weight loss; reduced appetite; dehydration; and feeling faint or fainting. Dry, bland foods and fluids together is the first line of treatment. Sometimes, medicines are prescribed to help nausea. Many women with HG have to be hospitalized.

Placenta Previa

Placenta previa occurs when the placenta covers part of or the entire opening of the cervix inside of the uterus. Symptoms include painless vaginal bleeding during second or third trimester. For some, there are no symptoms. If diagnosed after the 20th week of pregnancy, but with no bleeding, a woman will need to cut back on her activity level and increase bed rest. If bleeding is heavy, hospitalization may be needed.

Placental Abruption

Placental abruption occurs when the placenta separates from the uterine wall before delivery, which can mean the fetus doesn't get enough oxygen. Symptoms include vaginal bleeding, cramping, abdominal pain, and uterine tenderness. When the separation is minor, bed rest for a few days usually stops the bleeding. Moderate cases may require complete bed rest. Severe cases can require immediate medical attention and early delivery of the baby.

Preeclampsia

Preeclampsia is a condition starting after 20 weeks of pregnancy that causes high blood pressure and problems with the kidneys and other organs. Also called toxemia. Symptoms include high blood pressure; swelling of hands and face; too much protein in urine; stomach pain; blurred vision; dizziness; and headaches. The only cure is delivery, which may not be best for the baby.

Preterm Labor

Preterm labor is going into labor before 37 weeks of pregnancy. Medicines can stop labor from progressing. Bed rest is often advised. Sometimes, a woman must deliver early. Giving birth before 37 weeks is called preterm birth.

Infections During Pregnancy

During pregnancy, your baby is protected from many illnesses, like the common cold or a passing stomach bug. But some infections can be harmful to your pregnancy, your baby, or both. Easy steps, such as hand washing, practicing safe sex, and avoiding certain foods, can help protect you from some infections.

Bacterial Vaginosis (BV)

BV is a vaginal infection that is caused by an overgrowth of bacteria normally found in the vagina. Symptoms include grey or whitish discharge that has a foul, fishy odor and burning when passing urine or itching. Some women have no symptoms. BV is not passed through sexual contact, although it is linked with having a new or more than one sex partner. Women with symptoms should be tested for BV; antibiotics are used to treat it.

Group B Strep (GBS)

Group B strep is a type of bacteria often found in the vagina and rectum of healthy women; there are no symptoms. GBS usually is not harmful to you, but can be deadly to your baby if passed during childbirth. You can keep from passing GBS to your baby by getting tested at 35 to 37 weeks. If you have GBS, an antibiotic given to you during labor will protect your baby from infection.

Hepatitis B Virus (HBV)

HBV is a viral infection that can be passed to baby during birth. A vaccine can keep newborns from getting HBV. There may be no symptoms, or symptoms can include: nausea, vomiting, and diarrhea; dark urine and pale bowel movements; whites of eyes or skin looks yellow. Lab tests can find out if the mother is a carrier of hepatitis B.

Influenza (Flu)

Flu is a common viral infection that is more likely to cause severe illness in pregnant women than in women who are not pregnant. Pregnant woman with flu also have a greater chance for serious problems for their unborn baby, including premature labor and delivery. Symptoms include fever (sometimes) or feeling feverish/chills; cough; sore throat; runny or stuffy nose; muscle or body aches; headaches; feeling tired; vomiting and diarrhea (sometimes). Getting a flu shot is the first and most important step in protecting against flu.

It's A Fact!

You can protect your baby for life from HBV with the hepatitis B vaccine, which is a series of three shots.

Quick Tip

If you get sick with flu-like symptoms call your doctor right away. If needed, the doctor will prescribe an antiviral medicine that treats the flu.

Listeriosis

Listeriosis is an infection with the harmful bacteria called listeria. It is found in some refrigerated and ready-to-eat foods. Infection can cause early delivery or miscarriage. Symptoms include: fever, muscle aches, chills; sometimes diarrhea or nausea. If it progresses, severe headache and stiff neck can result. Avoid foods that can harbor listeria. Antibiotics are used to treat listeriosis.

Sexually Transmitted Infection (STI)

An STI is an infection that is passed through sexual contact. Many STIs can be passed to the baby in the womb or during birth. Symptoms depend on the STI. Often, a woman has no symptoms, which is why screening for STIs during pregnancy is so important. Treatments vary depending on the STI. Many STIs are treated easily with antibiotics.

Toxoplasmosis

This infection is caused by a parasite, which is found in cat feces, soil, and raw or undercooked meat. If passed to an unborn baby, the infection can cause hearing loss, blindness, or intellectual disabilities. You may have mild flu-like symptoms, or possibly no symptoms. You can lower your risk by: washing hands with soap after touching soil or raw meat; washing produce before eating; cooking meat completely; washing cooking utensils with hot, soapy water; and not cleaning cats' litter boxes. Medicines are used to treat a pregnant woman and her unborn baby.

It's A Fact!

STIs can be prevented by practicing safe sex. A woman can keep from passing an STI to her baby by being screened early in pregnancy.

Urinary Tract Infection (UTI)

A UTI is a bacterial infection in the urinary tract. If untreated, it can spread to the kidneys, which can cause preterm labor. Symptoms include: pain or burning when urinating; frequent urination; pelvis, back, stomach, or side pain; shaking, chills, fever, sweats. UTIs are treated with antibiotics.

Yeast Infection

A yeast infection is an infection caused by an overgrowth of bacteria normally found in the vagina. Yeast infections are more common during pregnancy than in other times of a woman's life. They do not threaten the health of your baby. But they can be uncomfortable and difficult to treat in pregnancy. Symptoms include: extreme itchiness in and around the vagina; burning, redness, and swelling of the vagina and the vulva; pain when passing urine or during sex; a thick, white vaginal discharge that looks like cottage cheese and does not have a bad smell. Vaginal creams and suppositories are used to treat yeast infection during pregnancy.

When To Call The Doctor

When you are pregnant don't wait to call your doctor or midwife if something is bothering or worrying you. Sometimes physical changes can be signs of a problem.

Call your doctor or midwife as soon as you can if you have any of the following:

- Bleeding or leaking fluid from the vagina
- Sudden or severe swelling in the face, hands, or fingers
- Severe or long-lasting headaches
- Discomfort, pain, or cramping in the lower abdomen
- Fever or chills
- Vomiting or persistent nausea
- Discomfort, pain, or burning with urination
- Problems seeing or blurred vision
- Feel dizzy
- Suspect your baby is moving less than normal after 28 weeks of pregnancy (If you count less than 10 movements within two hours.)
- Thoughts of harming yourself or your baby

Chapter 33

Anemia During Pregnancy

Anemia occurs when the number or size of a person's red blood cells are too low. Red blood cells are important because they carry oxygen from your lungs to all parts of your body. Without enough oxygen, your body cannot work as well as it should, and you feel tired and run down.

Anemia can affect anyone, but women are at greater risk for this condition. In women, iron and red blood cells are lost when bleeding occurs from very heavy or long periods (menstruation).

Anemia is common in pregnancy because a woman needs to have enough red blood cells to carry oxygen around her body and to her baby. So it's important for women to prevent anemia before, during, and after pregnancy. Women will probably be tested for anemia at least twice during pregnancy: during the first prenatal visit and then again between 24 and 28 weeks.

Causes Of Anemia

Iron Deficiency

Usually, a woman becomes anemic (has anemia) because her body isn't getting enough iron. Iron is a mineral that helps to create red blood cells. About half of all pregnant women don't have enough iron in their body (iron deficiency). In pregnancy, iron deficiency has been linked to an increased risk of preterm birth and low birthweight.

About This Chapter: Information in this chapter is from "Anemia," © 2009 March of Dimes Birth Defects Foundation. All rights reserved. For additional information, contact the March of Dimes at their website www .marchofdimes.com.

Illness Or Disease

Some women may have an illness that causes anemia. Diseases such as sickle cell anemia or thalassemia affect the quality and number of red blood cells the body produces. If you have a disease that causes anemia, talk with your health provider about how to treat anemia.

Signs Of Anemia

Anemia takes some time to develop. In the beginning, you may not have any signs or they may be mild. But as it gets worse, you may have these symptoms:

- Fatigue (very common)
- Weakness (very common)
- Dizziness
- Headache
- Numbness or coldness in your hands and feet
- Low body temperature
- Pale skin
- Rapid or irregular heartbeat
- Shortness of breath
- Chest pain
- Irritability
- Not doing well at work or in school

Because your heart has to work harder to pump more oxygen-rich blood through the body, all of these signs and symptoms can occur.

Quick Tip

Foods containing vitamin C can increase the amount of iron your body absorbs. So it's a good idea to include products such as orange juice, tomatoes, strawberries, and grapefruit in your daily diet.

Coffee, tea, egg yolks, milk, fiber, and soy protein can block your body from absorbing iron. Try to avoid these when eating iron-rich foods.

Getting Enough Iron

Before getting pregnant, women should get about 18 milligrams (mg) of iron per day. During pregnancy, the amount of iron you need jumps to 27 mg per day. Most pregnant women get this amount from eating foods that contain iron and taking prenatal vitamins that contain iron. Some women need to take iron supplements to prevent iron deficiency.

Iron-Rich Foods

You can help lower your risk of anemia by eating foods that contain iron during your entire pregnancy. These foods include:

- Poultry (dark meat)
- Dried fruits (apricots, prunes, figs, raisins, dates)
- Iron-fortified cereals, breads, and pastas
- Oatmeal
- Whole grains
- Blackstrap molasses
- Liver and other meats
- Seafood (learn about the safe kinds of seafood you can eat during pregnancy)
- Spinach, broccoli, kale, and other dark green leafy vegetables
- Baked potato with skin
- Beans and peas
- Nuts and seeds

Iron Supplements

If you are anemic, your health care provider may prescribe an iron supplement. Some iron supplements may cause heartburn, constipation, or nausea. Here are some tips to avoid or reduce these problems:

- Take the pills with meals.
- Start with small doses and work your way up to the full dose slowly. For example, try taking one pill a day for a few days, then two pills until you aren't bothered by that

amount. Increase the number of pills until you're taking the amount your health care provider recommends.

- Try different brands to see which works best for you. Be sure to discuss any changes with your health care provider ahead of time.

- Avoid taking iron pills at bedtime.

- Reduce constipation by drinking more water and by eating more fiber. Fiber is found in whole grain foods, breakfast cereals, fruits, and vegetables.

Chapter 34

Preeclampsia

High Blood Pressure In Pregnancy

Preeclampsia (pre-e-CLAMP-si-a) is one of the most common complications of pregnancy, impacting both the mother and the unborn baby. Affecting at least five to eight percent of all pregnancies, it is diagnosed by high blood pressure and the presence of protein in the urine, which is why the mother's blood pressure and urine are checked at every prenatal appointment. Most cases are very mild, occurring near term with healthy outcomes. It can, however, be very dangerous for mother and baby, progressing quite rapidly in some instances. It should be diagnosed early and managed closely to keep you and your baby safe. Here are some of the most frequently asked questions, but a more complete list and longer answers can be found at www.preeclampsia.org.

So What Is "Toxemia"?

You may encounter other names like toxemia, PET (pre-eclampsia/toxemia), PIH (pregnancy induced hypertension), and EPH gestosis (edema, proteinuria, hypertension), but these designations are all outdated terms and no longer used by medical experts.

How Is Preeclampsia Related To Eclampsia Or HELLP Syndrome?

Eclampsia and HELLP syndrome are other variations of preeclampsia. Seizures are the defining characteristic of eclampsia, which usually occur as a later complication of severe preeclampsia, but may also arise without any prior signs of severe disease. HELLP syndrome is one of the most severe forms of preeclampsia and occurs in about 15 percent of preeclamptic patients. It is

About This Chapter: Information in this chapter is from "Preeclampsia: Know the symptoms. Trust yourself," © 2010 Preeclampsia Foundation. All rights reserved. Reprinted with permission. The Preeclampsia Foundation is a 501(c) (3) nonprofit organization whose mission is to provide patient support and education, raise public awareness, catalyze research, and improve health care practices. For more information, visit www.preeclampsia.org.

sometimes mistaken for the flu or gall bladder problems. HELLP syndrome can lead to substantial injury to the mother's liver, a breakdown of her red blood cells, and lowered platelet count.

What Causes Preeclampsia? Can It Be Prevented?

The cause of preeclampsia remains unknown and, therefore, there is no sure way to prevent it. Numerous proposed theories have led to various attempts at prevention strategies, none of which have proven to be overwhelmingly successful. Baby aspirin, calcium, and other interventions have been studied and may be helpful in certain populations, but the results do not support widespread adoption in the U.S. There is, however, general agreement that the placenta plays a key role in preeclampsia, and that women with chronic hypertension and other risk factors are more susceptible. It is important to know the warning signs, trust yourself, attend prenatal visits, and have a strong partnership with your health care providers. Report your symptoms to them, ask questions, be persistent, and follow through.

When Can I Get Preeclampsia?

Preeclampsia can appear at any time during pregnancy, delivery, and up to six weeks postpartum, though it most frequently occurs late in the second or during the final trimester and resolves within 48 hours of delivery. Nonetheless, you should watch for symptoms even after delivery. Preeclampsia can develop gradually, or come on quite suddenly, even flaring up in a matter of hours, though the signs and symptoms may have gone undetected for weeks or months.

What Are The Symptoms Of Preeclampsia?

Preeclampsia can be particularly dangerous because many women have no symptoms until they are very sick or may ignore symptoms that resemble the "normal" effects of pregnancy on your body. See the list of signs and symptoms later in this chapter.

Who Gets Preeclampsia?

As many as one in every 12 pregnant women develop preeclampsia, including many who have no known risk factors. Some risk factors have been identified for increasing your chance of developing preeclampsia. Obesity, for example, is one risk factor that is perhaps modifiable. See the list of risk factors later in this chapter.

Is Preeclampsia Dangerous To The Mother?

Preeclampsia can cause your blood pressure to rise and put you at risk of brain injury. It can impair kidney and liver function, cause blood clotting problems, fluid to collect in the lungs, seizures and, in severe forms or left untreated, death. Maternal death from preeclampsia is rare, but does happen even in high-income countries; however, it is a significant cause of illness and death globally for mothers and infants.

Signs And Symptoms

- High blood pressure. 140/90 or higher. A rise in the systolic (higher number) of 30 or more, or the diastolic (lower number) of 15 or more over your baseline might be cause for concern.

- Protein in your urine. 300 milligrams in a 24 hour collection or 1+ on the dipstick.

- Swelling in the hands, feet, or face, especially around the eyes, if an indentation is left when applying thumb pressure, or if it has occurred rather suddenly.

- Headaches that just won't go away, even after taking medications for them.

- Changes in vision, double vision, blurriness, flashing lights, or auras.

- Nausea late in pregnancy is not normal and could be cause for concern.

- Upper abdominal pain (epigastric) or chest pain, sometimes mistaken for indigestion, gall bladder pain, or the flu.

- Sudden weight gain of two pounds or more in one week.

- Breathlessness. Breathing with difficulty, gasping, or panting.

If you have one or more of these signs and symptoms, you should see your doctor or go to an emergency room immediately.

Risk Factors

Personal History

- First pregnancy
- Preeclampsia in a previous pregnancy
- Over 40 or under 18 years of age
- High blood pressure before pregnancy
- Diabetes before or during pregnancy
- Multiple gestations

- Obesity (BMI>30). Calculate BMI at www.nhlbisupport.com/bmi/
- Lupus or other autoimmune disorders
- Polycystic ovarian syndrome
- Large interval between pregnancies
- In vitro fertilization
- Sickle cell disease

Family History

- Preeclampsia on mother's or father's side of the family
- High blood pressure or heart disease
- Diabetes

Share your risk factors with your health care provider.

If You Have Preeclampsia

How Does It Affect My Baby?

Preeclampsia can cause intrauterine growth restriction (IUGR) where the baby does not receive enough oxygen and nutrients to grow normally, or it can cause abruption, where the placenta separates from the wall of the uterus before the baby is born. It is a leading cause of prematurity, as some babies will need to be delivered early (before 37 weeks). Risks to a premature baby include incomplete lung development and many other potential health problems.

How Is Preeclampsia Treated?

The only cure for preeclampsia begins with delivery of the baby. Many factors guide a health care provider's decision about how to manage preeclampsia and when to deliver, including the gestational age and health of the baby, overall health and age of the mother, and a careful assessment of how the disease is progressing. This includes monitoring blood pressure and assessing the results of laboratory tests that indicate the condition of the mother's kidneys, liver, or the ability of her blood to clot. Other tests monitor how well the unborn baby is growing and/or if he or she seems in danger. Treatments may include magnesium sulfate to prevent seizures and other medications to lower blood pressure. Sometimes a watch-and-wait approach may be used with or without medications, but if the mother or baby's health is in serious danger, delivery may be the only option. Steroid shots may be given to aid a preterm baby's lung development before delivery. Often, women with preeclampsia will stay in the hospital because the symptoms may suddenly worsen and close monitoring is necessary.

Do These Medications Pose A Threat To Me Or My Baby?

Blood pressure medications rarely cause any side effects in the mother and, if prescribed, it probably means your blood pressure is high enough to be a greater risk to you or your baby than the medications. Magnesium sulfate is generally safe for the baby, but may cause hot flashes, sweating, increased thirst, vision changes, sleepiness, mild confusion, muscle weakness, and shortness of breath in the mother. These side effects should all disappear when the medication is stopped.

Can I Stay At Home On Bed Rest?

Sometimes, women with mild preeclampsia will be put on home bed rest. In this case, you will probably need to have frequent visits with your health care provider, and blood and urine testing to be sure the condition is not getting worse. The well-being of your baby will be checked frequently with heart monitoring and ultrasounds. If you are prescribed home bed rest, always be alert for any symptoms because preeclampsia can change rapidly.

Will I Get It Again?

Various experts suggest your chances of getting it again range from five to 80 percent, depending on when you had preeclampsia in a prior pregnancy, how severe it was, and your general health at conception. Women with a history of preeclampsia should have a consultation with a high-risk pregnancy specialist prior to conception.

Chapter 35

Preterm Labor And Birth

Preterm birth is any birth that occurs before the 37th week of pregnancy. It is the cause of many infant deaths and lingering infant illnesses in the United States. Every pregnant woman needs to know about preterm labor and birth—why it happens and what she can do to help prevent it.

Preterm birth occurs in about 12 percent of all pregnancies in the United States, often for reasons we just don't understand. A normal pregnancy should last about 40 weeks. That amount of time gives the baby the best chance to be healthy. A pregnancy that ends between 20 weeks and 37 weeks is considered preterm, and all preterm babies are at significant risk for health problems. The earlier the birth, the greater the risk.

You might have read in the newspapers about babies who are born really early and do very well. But it's important for you to know that those babies are the exceptions. Babies who are born very preterm are at a very high risk for brain problems, breathing problems, digestive problems, and death in the first few days of life. Unfortunately, they also are at risk for problems later in their lives in the form of delayed development and learning problems in school. The effects of premature birth can be devastating throughout the child's life. The earlier in pregnancy a baby is born, the more health problems it is likely to have.

Why Preterm Labor Occurs

There are no easy answers. Stress might play a part for some women, personal health history or infection for others, or smoking or drug use for others. With funding from the March

About This Chapter: Information in this chapter is from "Preterm labor and birth: A serious pregnancy complication," © 2010 March of Dimes Birth Defects Foundation. All rights reserved. For additional information, contact the March of Dimes at their website www.marchofdimes.com.

of Dimes and others, researchers are studying how various factors contribute to the complex problem of premature labor and birth.

Women At Risk For Preterm Labor

Preterm labor and delivery can happen to any pregnant woman. But they happen more often to some women than to others. Researchers continue to study preterm labor and birth. They have identified some risk factors, but still cannot generally predict which women will give birth too early. Having a risk factor does not mean a woman will have preterm labor or preterm birth. It just means that she is at greater risk than other women.

Three groups of women are at greatest risk of preterm labor and birth:

1. Women who have had a previous preterm birth

2. Women who are pregnant with twins, triplets, or more

3. Women with certain uterine or cervical abnormalities

If you have any of these three risk factors, it's especially important for you to know the signs and symptoms of preterm labor and what to do if they occur.

Lifestyle And Environmental Risks

Some studies have found that certain lifestyle and environmental factors may put a woman at greater risk of preterm labor. These factors include:

- Late or no prenatal care

- Smoking

- Drinking alcohol

- Using illegal drugs

- Exposure to the medication DES

- Domestic violence, including physical, sexual, or emotional abuse

- Lack of social support

- Stress

- Long working hours with long periods of standing

- Exposure to certain environmental pollutants

Medical Risks

Certain medical conditions during pregnancy may increase the likelihood that a woman will have preterm labor. These conditions include:

- Urinary tract infections, vaginal infections, sexually transmitted infections, and possibly other infections

- Diabetes

- High blood pressure and preeclampsia

- Clotting disorders (thrombophilia)

- Bleeding from the vagina

- Certain birth defects in the baby

- Being pregnant with a single fetus that is the result of in vitro fertilization (IVF)

- Being underweight before pregnancy

- Obesity

- Short time period between pregnancies (less than six to nine months between birth and the beginning of the next pregnancy)

Groups At Increased Risk

Researchers have also identified certain groups that are at increased risk of having a premature baby. These groups include:

- African-American women

- Women younger than 17 and older than 35

- Women who have a low income

Preventing Preterm Labor And Birth

You can help prevent preterm birth by learning the symptoms of preterm labor and following some simple instructions. The first thing to do is to get medical care both before and during pregnancy. If you do have preterm labor, get medical help quickly. This will improve the chances that you and your baby will do well.

Medications sometimes slow or stop labor if they are given early enough. Drugs called corticosteroids, if given 24 hours before birth, can help the baby's lungs and brain mature. This can prevent some of the worst health problems a preterm baby has. Only if a woman receives medical care quickly can drugs be helpful. Knowing what to look for is essential.

> **It's A Fact!**
>
> Treatment with a form of the hormone progesterone may help prevent premature birth in some women who have already had a premature baby.

Symptoms Of Preterm Labor

Remember, preterm labor is any labor that occurs between 20 weeks and 37 weeks of pregnancy. Here are the symptoms:

- Contractions (your abdomen tightens like a fist) every 10 minutes or more often
- Change in vaginal discharge (leaking fluid or bleeding from your vagina)
- Pelvic pressure—the feeling that your baby is pushing down
- Low, dull backache
- Cramps that feel like your period
- Abdominal cramps with or without diarrhea

If you start to have any of these symptoms between 20 weeks and 37 weeks of pregnancy, follow the instructions in the section "What to do if you have symptoms of preterm labor."

Don't let anyone tell you that these symptoms are "normal discomforts of pregnancy." If any of them (you don't need to have all of them) happen before your 37th week of pregnancy, you need to do something about it.

What To Do If You Have Symptoms Of Preterm Labor

Call your health care provider or go to the hospital right away if you think you are having preterm labor. Your provider may tell you to:

- Come to the office or go to the hospital for evaluation.
- Stop what you are doing and rest on your left side for one hour.

- Drink two to three glasses of water or juice (not coffee or soda).

If the symptoms get worse, or don't go away after one hour, call your health care provider again or go to the hospital. If the symptoms go away, take it easy for the rest of the day. If the symptoms stop but come back, call your health care provider again or go to the hospital.

You and your health care provider are a team, working together to have a healthy pregnancy and healthy baby. Your team works best when both of you participate fully, so your knowledge about preterm labor can be essential in helping to prevent a preterm birth. Talk to your health care provider about all of this, and be sure to keep all of your prenatal care appointments. Preterm birth is one of the complications of pregnancy that health care providers are working hard to eliminate. Your participation in this effort is just as important as theirs!

Quick Tip

When you call your provider, be sure to tell the person on the phone that you are concerned about the possibility of preterm labor. The only way your provider can know if preterm labor is starting is by doing an internal examination of your cervix (the bottom of your uterus). If your cervix is opening up (dilating), preterm labor could be beginning.

Chapter 36

Managing Asthma And Allergies During Pregnancy

If you have asthma or allergies and are pregnant or considering becoming pregnant, this important information will promote a safe pregnancy and delivery, and a healthy baby.

Asthma affects almost seven percent of pregnant women and can cause serious complications for both mother and child if not controlled properly during pregnancy. Complications for the expectant mother may include high blood pressure and preeclampsia, a disorder that occurs when high blood pressure is accompanied by fluid retention and leaking of protein into the mother's urine, potentially damaging her kidneys, brain, liver, and eyes. If the condition results in seizures, it can be deadly for both the mother and baby. Other complications for the baby include an increased risk of premature birth, low birth weight, slow growth, and stillbirth.

The good news is that asthma and allergies can be controlled, and when they are, the risks to mother and baby are extremely low.

This chapter discusses how to safely control your asthma and allergies while you await the birth of your baby, and answers several questions you might have.

How will my pregnancy affect the severity of my asthma?

If you have asthma, you probably feel a tightness in your chest and may experience wheezing, shortness of breath, and/or coughing. These symptoms are caused by muscle spasms that constrict the flow of air to the lungs. The linings of the airways become inflamed and swollen, and may be clogged by excess mucus. Asthma may be triggered by allergens, including pollen, mold, animal dander, house dust mites, and cockroaches; other environmental factors; exercise; infections; and stress.

Your asthma may become worse during your pregnancy, especially if your condition is considered severe. On the other hand, about a third of asthma patients improve during pregnancy, especially if their disease was mild before they became pregnant. Another third experience no change. If your asthma or asthma attacks become worse, it will most likely occur during 24 to 36 weeks of your pregnancy. Only about one in 10 women with asthma have symptoms during delivery.

The hormonal changes that occur during your pregnancy may affect your nose, sinuses, and lungs, causing congestion and shortness of breath. Your doctor will help you determine if these symptoms, which may be confused with your asthma or may trigger your asthma, are actually caused by the disease.

If you've been pregnant before, you can probably expect your asthma to behave the same way in subsequent pregnancies. Within three months of your baby's birth, your asthma probably will return to the way it was before you became pregnant.

How will I know if my asthma is affecting my baby?

Depending on your age and any other risk factors, your doctor may conduct several tests throughout your pregnancy to monitor and evaluate your asthma and the effect it has on you and your baby's health.

Sonography or ultrasound can be performed during the first trimester to confirm the accuracy of your estimated due date. The test may be repeated later if slow growth in the baby is suspected.

Electronic heart rate monitoring, called "non-stress testing" or "contraction-stress testing," and ultrasound may be used in the third trimester to assess your baby's well-being. If you are experiencing significant asthma symptoms during this trimester, the frequency of the monitoring may be increased. All asthma patients should record their baby's activity and kick counts daily to help monitor the baby, according to their doctor's instructions.

If you experience a severe asthma attack during your pregnancy in which your symptoms do not quickly improve, there is a risk you may experience hypoxemia, or a low oxygen state. This is an important time to assess your baby's health, and continuous electronic fetal heart rate monitoring may be necessary, along with measurements of your lung function.

Fortunately, the majority of asthma patients do well during labor and delivery, although careful fetal monitoring remains very important. If you are a low-risk patient with well-controlled asthma, a fetal assessment can be accomplished by 20 minutes of electronic monitoring shortly after you are admitted to the hospital.

If you have severe asthma or other risk factors, more intensive fetal monitoring and observation is recommended.

What steps can I take to control my asthma and allergies while I'm pregnant?

Asthma and allergies are often connected. Most asthma patients are allergic to one or more allergens such as pollens, molds, pet dander, house dust mites, and cockroaches. These allergens may trigger your asthma symptoms or make existing symptoms worse.

Other non-allergic substances also may worsen your asthma and allergies. These include tobacco smoke, paint and chemical fumes, strong odors, environmental pollutants (including ozone and smog) and drugs, such as aspirin or beta-blockers (used to treat high blood pressure, migraine headaches, and heart disorders).

By avoiding specific triggers, you can decrease the frequency and intensity of your asthma and allergy symptoms. If a patient tests allergic to a specific trigger, allergists-immunologists recommend the following avoidance steps:

- Remove allergy-causing pets from the house.

- Seal pillows, mattresses, and box springs in special dust mite-proof casings (your allergist should be able to give you information regarding comfortable cases).

- Wash bedding weekly in 130 degrees F water (comforters may be dry-cleaned periodically) to kill dust mites. Keep home humidity under 50 percent to control dust mite and mold growth.

- Use filtering vacuums or "filter vacuum bags" to control airborne dust when cleaning.

- Close windows, use air-conditioning, and avoid outdoor activity between 5 a.m. and 10 a.m., when pollen and pollution are at their highest.

Can I use my asthma and allergy medications while I'm pregnant and nursing?

Today there are many excellent medications for treating asthma and allergies. Although no medication can be proven entirely safe for use during pregnancy, you and your doctor will work together to develop a treatment plan that carefully balances medication use and symptom control, and assures that the potential benefits of the medication outweigh the potential risks of the medication and of uncontrolled asthma.

Since the symptoms associated with asthma and allergies can vary from day to day, month to month, or season to season, regardless of pregnancy, your treatment plan will be based on the severity of your disease and previous experience using specific medications during pregnancy.

It's important to remember that the use of medication should not replace the avoidance of the allergens or irritants that trigger your asthma and allergies, since avoidance can potentially reduce your need for medication.

In general, the same medications used during pregnancy are appropriate during labor and delivery and when nursing. To obtain the lowest concentration of a medication in breast milk, it is recommended that you take the medication 15 minutes after nursing or three to four hours before your baby's next feeding.

Can I receive allergy shots or a flu shot when I'm pregnant?

Allergy shots (immunotherapy) are often effective if you continue to experience symptoms despite allergen avoidance and proper medication. If you currently are receiving immuno-therapy for the treatment of your asthma and/or allergies, it can be carefully continued during pregnancy if you benefit from the treatment and do not experience any adverse reactions. It is not recommended, however, that immunotherapy be initiated during a pregnancy.

If you have moderate or severe asthma, an influenza (flu) vaccine is recommended. There is no evidence of risk for you or your baby.

It's A Fact!

Medications used during pregnancy are usually selected based on the following criteria:

- Inhaled medications are generally preferred because they have a more localized effect with only small amounts entering the bloodstream.
- Time-tested older medications are preferred since there is more experience with their use during pregnancy.
- Medication use is limited in the first trimester as much as possible when the baby is developing the most, although birth defects due to medications are rare (no more than one percent of all birth defects are attributable to all medications).

Chapter 37

If You Are Pregnant And Diabetic

Diabetes is a condition in which your body cannot use sugars and starches (carbohydrates) from food to make energy. As a result, your body collects extra sugar in your blood. The extra sugar can lead to heart, eye, and kidney damage. If you are pregnant, the extra sugar increases the chances for problems with your baby, including birth defects.

Diabetes that occurs before pregnancy can be either type 1 or type 2.

Diabetes Can Harm You And Your Baby

A woman who does not have control of her diabetes and gets pregnant has a greater chance of having a baby with a birth defect than a woman without diabetes.

Diabetes that is not controlled can do the following:

- Cause your baby to have serious birth defects. If your blood sugar is out of control, it can lead to health problems and serious birth defects, such as those of your baby's brain, spine, and heart.

- Increase your chances for stillbirth or miscarriage.

- Cause your baby to be born early. A baby born too early can have breathing problems, heart problems, bleeding into the brain, intestinal problems, or vision problems.

- Make your baby grow very large (weigh more than nine pounds), which in turn can lead to problems with the delivery for you and your baby. A large baby born through the birth

About This Chapter: Information in this chapter is from "Got diabetes? Thinking about having a baby?" a publication of the Centers for Disease Control and Prevention, 2010.

canal can injure nerves in his shoulder; break her collarbone; or, rarely, have brain damage from lack of oxygen. You might have to have a cesarean section (an operation to get the baby out through your abdomen), which usually means a longer recovery time for you after your baby is born.

- Cause your newborn to have quickly changing blood sugars after delivery. Your baby's doctor will watch your baby for low blood sugar after birth and treat it if needed.

Other problems that sometimes happen with diabetes include the following:

- You may also develop preeclampsia. This means you have protein in your urine and high blood pressure. Preeclampsia can harm you by causing you to have seizures or a stroke. It also might cause your baby to be born early.

- Very large babies are more likely to become overweight or obese during childhood and adolescence. Such obesity can lead to type 2 diabetes.

- Controlling your diabetes before and during your pregnancy will help prevent such problems as birth defects, prematurity, miscarriage, and stillbirth. If you find that you are pregnant before your diabetes is controlled, taking steps now to control your blood sugar is the best way to care for your baby.

Quick Tip

If you are diabetic, it is best to plan a pregnancy. If you find that you are pregnant before your blood sugar is under control, the best way to care for your baby is to start now to control your blood sugar. Talk with your doctor to learn how.

Have A Healthy Pregnancy And A Healthy Baby

You can do the following things to help:

1. Eat healthy foods and stay active

   - Work with a dietitian or diabetes educator to develop a diabetes meal plan for yourself. Learn what to eat to keep your blood sugar under control.

   - Stay active to help keep your blood sugar under control. Exercise regularly—before, during, and after pregnancy. Moderate exercise, such as a brisk walk, 30 minutes a day, five days a week is a good goal if your doctor is okay with it.

2. Take your medicines.

- Follow your doctor's advice.

- Take your medicines as directed, including insulin if ordered by your doctor.

3. Monitor your blood sugar often

- Be aware that your blood sugar can change very quickly, becoming too high or too low. What you eat, how much you exercise, and your growing baby will change your blood sugar many times during the day.

- Check your blood sugar often—as directed by your doctor any time you have symptoms.

- Know what blood sugar levels mean. Learn how to adjust what you eat; how much you exercise; and, if prescribed, how much insulin to take depending on your blood sugar tests.

4. Control and treat low blood sugar quickly

- Check your blood sugar right away if you have symptoms.

- Treat low blood sugar quickly. Always carry with you a quick source of sugar, like hard candy or glucose tablets.

- Wear a medical alert diabetes bracelet.

It's A Fact!

Insulin is usually made in the body and helps change sugars and starches into energy. If the body doesn't make enough insulin or can't use the insulin it makes, extra insulin is given in a shot.

Stay Healthy After The Birth Of Your Baby

Take care of yourself as you begin to take care of your baby:

- Monitor and control your blood sugar.

- See your doctor regularly. Usually twice a year, your doctor will check your A1C (a blood test that shows how well your blood sugar has been controlled during the past three months).

- Take your medicines.

- Control and treat low blood sugar quickly.

- Continue to eat healthy foods.

- Stay active. Exercise 30 minutes a day five days a week.

- Talk with your doctor about your plans for more children BEFORE your next pregnancy.

- Watch your weight. Six to twelve months after your baby is born, your weight should be back down to what you weighed before you got pregnant. If you still weigh too much, work to lose five percent to seven percent (10 to 14 pounds if you weigh 200 pounds) of your body weight.

- Plan to lose your weight slowly. This will help you keep it off.

Chapter 38

Gestational Diabetes

Gestational diabetes is diabetes that a woman can develop during pregnancy.

When you have diabetes, your body cannot use the sugars and starches (carbohydrates) it takes in as food to make energy. As a result, your body collects extra sugar in your blood.

We don't know all the causes of gestational diabetes. Some—but not all—women with gestational diabetes are overweight before getting pregnant or have diabetes in the family. From one in 50 to one in 20 pregnant women has gestational diabetes. It is more common in Native American, Alaskan Native, Hispanic, Asian, and Black women, but it is found in White women, too.

Gestational Diabetes Can Affect Your Baby

Gestational diabetes that is not controlled can cause your baby to have the following problems:

- Grow very large (weigh more than nine pounds), which in turn can lead to problems with the delivery of your baby. A large baby born through the birth canal can injure nerves in his shoulder; break her collarbone; or, rarely, have brain damage from lack of oxygen.

- Have quickly changing blood sugar after delivery. Your baby's doctor will watch for low blood sugar after birth and treat it if needed.

- Be more likely to become overweight or obese during childhood or adolescence. Obesity can lead to type 2 diabetes.

About This Chapter: Information in this chapter is from "Diabetes and Pregnancy: Gestational Diabetes," a publication of the Centers for Disease Control and Prevention, January 2011.

> **It's A Fact!**
>
> Gestational diabetes can be controlled.
>
> Work with your doctor to make a plan to keep your blood sugar in control. Following this plan can help you have a healthy pregnancy and baby. It also can help you and your baby stay healthy after birth.

Gestational Diabetes Can Affect You

Gestational diabetes that is not controlled can cause you to have the following problems:

- Have problems during delivery.

- Have a very large baby and need to have a cesarean section (c-section) (an operation to get your baby out through your abdomen).

- Take longer to recover from childbirth if your baby is delivered by c-section.

Other problems that sometimes happen with gestational diabetes include the following:

- Women with gestational diabetes also can develop preeclampsia.

- Sometimes, diabetes does not go away after delivery or comes back later after pregnancy. When this happens, the diabetes then is called type 2 diabetes.

Work with your doctor before, during, and after pregnancy to prevent problems.

> **What's It Mean?**
>
> **Preeclampsia:** Preeclampsia is a problem that develops in some women during pregnancy. Women with preeclampsia have high blood pressure; protein in their urine; and, often, swollen feet, legs, fingers, and hands. Preeclampsia can harm you by causing seizures or a stroke. It might also cause your baby to be born early.
>
> **Type 2 Diabetes:** Type 2 diabetes is a condition in which the body either makes too little insulin or can't use the insulin it makes to use blood sugar for energy. Often, type 2 diabetes can be controlled through eating a proper diet, exercising regularly, and keeping a healthy weight. Some people with type 2 diabetes have to take diabetes pills or insulin, or both.

Now Is The Time To Keep You And Your Baby Healthy

It is important during your pregnancy to keep your blood sugar under control. Here's how:

1. See your doctor regularly.

    *   Ask your doctor if you need to see him or her more often because of your diabetes.

    *   Work with your doctor and, together, you will be able to catch problems early, or even prevent them entirely.

2. Eat healthy foods and stay active.

    *   Work with a dietitian or diabetes educator to develop a diabetes meal plan for yourself. Learn what to eat to keep your blood sugar under control.

    *   Stay active to help keep your blood sugar under control. Exercise regularly—before, during, and after pregnancy. Moderate exercise, such as a brisk walk, 30 minutes a day, five days a week is a good goal if it is okay with your doctor.

3. Take your medicines.

    *   Follow your doctor's advice.

    *   Take your medicines as directed.

4. Monitor your blood sugar often.

    *   Be aware that your blood sugar can change very quickly, becoming too high or too low. What you eat, how much you exercise, and your growing baby will change your blood sugar many times during the day.

    *   Check your blood sugar often—as directed by your doctor, and any time you have symptoms.

    *   Know what blood sugar levels mean. Learn how to adjust what you eat; how much you exercise; and, if prescribed, how much insulin to take depending on your blood sugar tests.

5. Control and treat low blood sugar quickly.

    *   Check your blood sugar right away if you have symptoms.

    *   Treat low blood sugar quickly. Always carry with you a quick source of sugar, like hard candy or glucose tablets.

    *   Wear a medical alert diabetes bracelet.

> **It's A Fact!**
> Insulin is usually made in the body and helps change sugars and starches into energy. If the body doesn't make enough insulin or can't use the insulin it makes, extra insulin is given in a shot.

Stay Healthy After The Birth Of Your Baby

Gestational diabetes goes away after pregnancy, but sometimes diabetes stays. It's important to be checked for diabetes after your baby is born. About half of all women who have gestational diabetes get type 2 diabetes later in life.

After pregnancy and in the future, do the following:

- Make sure to ask your doctor about testing for diabetes soon after delivery and again six weeks after delivery.

- Continue to eat healthy foods and exercise regularly.

- Have regular checkups and get your blood sugar checked by your doctor every one to three years.

- Talk with your doctor about your plans for more children before your next pregnancy.

- Watch your weight. Six to twelve months after your baby is born, your weight should be back down to what you weighed before you got pregnant. If you still weigh too much, work to lose five percent to seven percent (10 to 14 pounds if you weigh 200 pounds) of your body weight.

- Plan to lose weight slowly. This will help you keep it off.

Eating healthy, losing weight, and exercising regularly can help you delay or prevent type 2 diabetes in the future. Talk with your doctor to learn more.

Chapter 39

Preparing For Multiple Births

Over the past two decades, there's been a phenomenal rise in the number of multiple births in the United States. Between 1980 and 2004, the number of twin births increased by 70 percent and the number of births involving three or more babies has quadrupled.

What's responsible for this dramatic rise in multiple births? And how should you prepare for your own multiple birth experience?

The Miracle Of Multiples

Several factors contribute to the development of a multiple pregnancy:

- **Heredity:** A history of multiple births on a woman's side of the family increases her chances of having a multiple pregnancy.

- **Race:** Women of African descent are the most likely to have multiple pregnancies.

- **Number Of Prior Pregnancies:** Having more than one previous pregnancy, especially a multiple pregnancy, increases the chance of having a multiple pregnancy.

- **Delayed Childbearing:** Older women who get pregnant are more likely to have multiples.

- **Infertility Treatment:** Fertility drugs, which stimulate the ovaries to release multiple eggs, or assisted reproductive technology (ART), which transfers multiple embryos into the womb (such as in vitro fertilization, or IVF), greatly increase a woman's chance of having a multiple pregnancy.

About This Chapter: Information in this chapter is from "Preparing For Multiple Births," November 2010, reprinted with permission from www.kidshealth.org. Copyright © 2010 The Nemours Foundation. This information was provided by KidsHealth, one of the largest resources online for medically reviewed health information written for parents, kids, and teens. For more articles like this one, visit www.KidsHealth.org, or www.TeensHealth.org.

It's the last two factors that have been on the rise in the last couple of decades and are probably responsible for the increase in multiple births.

The Types Of Multiples

There are two types of twins: monozygotic (identical) and dizygotic (fraternal).

Identical twins result from a single fertilized egg dividing into separate halves and continuing to develop into two separate but identical babies. These twins are genetically identical, with the same chromosomes and similar physical characteristics. They're the same sex and have the same blood type, hair, and eye color.

Fraternal twins come from two eggs that are fertilized by two separate sperm and are no more alike than other siblings born to the same parents. They may or may not be the same sex. This type of twins is much more common, and only this type is affected by heredity, maternal age, race, and number of prior pregnancies.

It's A Fact!

Supertwins is a common term for triplets and other higher-order multiple births, such as quadruplets or quintuplets. These babies can be identical, fraternal, or a combination of both. But higher-order births are rare; triplets occur in approximately one in 7,000 to 8,000 births, whereas quintuplets are likely to be born only once in 47 million births.

The Risks Of Multiple Births

The most immediate risk involved with multiple births is pre-term (or early) labor resulting in premature births. A typical, single pregnancy lasts about 40 weeks, but a twin pregnancy often lasts between 35 to 37 weeks. Nearly half of all twins are born prematurely (before 37 weeks), and the risk of having a premature delivery increases with higher-order multiples.

Premature babies (preemies) can have numerous health challenges. Because the care of premature babies is so different from that of full-term infants, preemies are usually placed in a neonatal intensive care unit (NICU) after delivery. The risk of developing health problems increases with the degree of prematurity—babies born closer to their due date have a lower risk.

In addition to the possibility of premature births, other medical conditions that are more likely to occur during a multiple pregnancy include preeclampsia, gestational diabetes, placental problems, and fetal growth problems. Being part of a multiple birth can also be associated with long-term health problems in the infants. Developmental delays and cerebral palsy occur more commonly in twins than in single births, and there's a higher risk of enduring health problems with higher-order multiple births.

Because of these concerns, many doctors who specialize in fertility treatments require prospective parents to undergo intensive counseling on the possibilities and risks associated with multiple births.

Staying Healthy During A Multiple Pregnancy

Eating properly, getting enough rest, and making regular trips to the doctor are critical measures for any expectant mother to stay healthy. And a woman with a multiple pregnancy might be scheduled for more frequent appointments with her obstetrician/gynecologist (OB-GYN) than a women who is pregnant with a single fetus.

The need for frequent, intensive prenatal care is of the utmost importance in a multiple pregnancy. You'll want to be particularly careful about finding health care professionals who have experience with multiple births. Because multiple pregnancies are automatically termed high-risk, the need for specialized health care is vital to ensuring that you and your babies receive the best care available.

Because you may not know anyone who has experienced a multiple birth, asking for a referral from a friend may not be productive. Instead, ask your doctor or OB-GYN to recommend a facility that specializes in multiple births. You should be part of a pre-term birth prevention program at your hospital and have immediate access to a specialized NICU should you go into early labor or if one of your babies is born with a health problem.

Your Nutrition

If you're pregnant with multiples, you should follow general pregnancy nutrition guidelines, including increasing your calcium and folic acid intake. Pregnant women need additional calcium, so extra milk or fortified orange juice, broccoli, sardines, or other calcium-rich foods should be added to your diet.

As with all expectant mothers, folic acid is extremely important. Taking folic acid one month prior to and throughout the first three months of pregnancy will decrease the risk of neural tube defects (such as spina bifida).

Another dietary requirement that needs to be increased if you're expecting more than one baby is protein, which has several important functions. First, proteins serve as the building materials of body tissue. They also act as enzymes that regulate chemical reactions to keep a body growing and functioning.

During pregnancy, an increased supply of iron is also needed for hemoglobin, the substance in red blood cells that binds oxygen for delivery to the tissues. Insufficient iron can lead to a condition known as iron-deficiency anemia. Anemia occurs when the number of healthy red blood cells decreases in the body, and is relatively common in multiple pregnancies. Anemia can cause a decreased appetite and extreme fatigue during a pregnancy, as well as a reduced oxygen supply to the developing babies. Your doctor will probably prescribe an iron supplement, as your requirement for this mineral usually can't be met by diet alone.

Additional fetuses also mean an increased need for all other nutrients (such as zinc, copper, vitamin C, and vitamin D). So it's important to take your prenatal vitamin supplement every day. But just because you're carrying more than one baby doesn't mean you should take more than one prenatal vitamin—one is enough and too much can even be harmful.

Quick Tip

Iron is absorbed more easily when combined with foods high in acid, such as yogurt, and those with high amounts of vitamin C, like orange juice.

Your Weight

Mothers carrying multiples are expected to gain more weight during pregnancy than mothers carrying a single fetus. But exactly how much weight you should gain depends on your prepregnancy weight and the number of fetuses, so make sure to talk to your doctor.

In general, though, you should consume about 300 additional calories a day for each fetus. It might be tough to eat a lot when your abdomen is full of babies, so try to eat smaller, more frequent meals.

Your Comfort

Of course, expecting multiples means that you're probably experiencing the typical discomforts of pregnancy more intensely. Nurturing yourself can help ease the stress of pregnancy.

Even a warm bath can help lift your spirits. (Just make sure you have someone around to help lift you out of the tub!)

Expectant partners can help, too. Something as simple as having someone brush your hair can make the discomforts of pregnancy fade momentarily. It helps, too, if your partner remembers that your body is going through tremendous hormonal changes. Communication and understanding can be the keys to truly enjoying this special time in your lives.

Preparing For Childbirth

Getting ready for a multiple birth may seem overwhelming, and concerns about pre-term labor can be additional burdens for you to bear. The best reassurance is knowing that you have a network of support around you: capable doctors, a caring hospital staff, and hopefully a supportive partner, family members, and/or friends.

To help you be more comfortable with the birth process as it unfolds, you should also discuss the options of vaginal delivery versus cesarean section (c-section) with your doctor well before your due date. Several factors affect the safety of each approach. Even if you and your doctor agree to attempt a vaginal delivery, circumstances may arise during labor or delivery that make a c-section necessary.

You may opt to have additional birthing attendants in the room during labor and birth. For example, midwives are becoming more common. Working in collaboration with a medical doctor, a certified nurse-midwife (CNM) has specialized training in midwifery and is registered or licensed in all 50 states.

Hiring a doula is another option. The term comes from ancient Greece, where the doula was the primary attendant to the female head of the household. Today, doulas offer support services to women during the birth, as well as after delivery, by assisting with infant care and household chores.

Special Delivery

As labor begins, you'll likely be connected to a fetal monitor so your doctor can check each baby's progress. The interval between the birth of each baby delivered vaginally is usually less than an hour. And here's one piece of good news: Because multiple-birth babies tend to be smaller than single ones, it's easier to push them out. Luckily, they only come out one at a time!

In the case of multiples, though, a vaginal delivery may not always be possible. The crowded uterus can cause compression of the placenta or umbilical cord of any of the soon-to-be-born babies during labor. Prolonged compression may put one or more babies at serious risk as labor progresses during attempts at vaginal delivery. So prompt delivery by c-section may be necessary in these cases.

Positioning of the babies can also affect the safety of a vaginal delivery. It's common for the first baby to be born head first, whereas the subsequent infants may be breech (buttocks or feet first), transverse (sideways), or head first when entering the birth canal. Usually, if the first fetus is not head first, the babies will be delivered by c-section. And most triplets and other higher-order multiples are born by c-section.

If your doctor needs to perform a c-section, a catheter will be placed in your bladder, you'll be given anesthesia, and an incision will be made in your abdomen and uterus. The doctor will then deliver your babies through the incision. The babies will be delivered within just a few minutes of each other with this approach.

Many babies born prematurely will need to go immediately to the NICU for the special care they need. Visitations by family members are usually encouraged, often right from the first day.

Quick Tip

If you go into labor prematurely, you and your unborn babies will be closely monitored for signs of distress. You may have to make decisions on the delivery method and procedures at this time, so consider your options before arriving at the hospital.

Taking Your Babies Home

The first days, weeks, and months are often the most difficult for parents of multiples, as everyone learns to get used to the frequent feedings, lack of sleep, and little personal time involved in parenting multiples.

Enlist whatever help you can get—from neighbors, family members, and friends—for household chores and daily tasks. Having extra hands around can not only make feedings easier and help you rest and recover from delivery, it can also give you the precious time you need to get to know your babies.

Chapter 40

Ectopic Pregnancy

An ectopic pregnancy is an abnormal pregnancy that occurs outside the womb (uterus). The baby (fetus) cannot survive, and often does not develop at all in this type of pregnancy.

Causes

An ectopic pregnancy occurs when a pregnancy starts outside the womb (uterus). The most common site for an ectopic pregnancy is within one of the tubes through which the egg passes from the ovary to the uterus (fallopian tube). However, in rare cases, ectopic pregnancies can occur in the ovary, stomach area, or cervix.

An ectopic pregnancy is often caused by a condition that blocks or slows the movement of a fertilized egg through the fallopian tube to the uterus. This may be caused by a physical blockage in the tube by hormonal factors and by other factors, such as smoking.

Most cases of scarring are caused by:

- Past ectopic pregnancy
- Past infection in the fallopian tubes
- Surgery of the fallopian tubes

Up to 50 percent of women who have ectopic pregnancies have had swelling (inflammation) of the fallopian tubes (salpingitis) or pelvic inflammatory disease (PID).

Some ectopic pregnancies can be due to:

- Birth defects of the fallopian tubes

- Complications of a ruptured appendix

- Endometriosis

- Scarring caused by previous pelvic surgery

The following may also increase the risk of ectopic pregnancy:

- Age over 35

- Having had many sexual partners

- In vitro fertilization

In a few cases, the cause is unknown.

> **It's A Fact!**
> Ectopic pregnancies occur in one in every 40 to one in every 100 pregnancies.

Sometimes, a woman will become pregnant after having her tubes tied (tubal sterilization). Ectopic pregnancies are more likely to occur two or more years after the procedure, rather than right after it. In the first year after sterilization, only about six percent of pregnancies will be ectopic, but most pregnancies that occur two to three years after tubal sterilization will be ectopic.

Ectopic pregnancy is also more likely in women who have:

- Had surgery to reverse tubal sterilization in order to become pregnant

- Had an intrauterine device (IUD) and became pregnant (very unlikely when IUDs are in place)

Symptoms

- Abnormal vaginal bleeding

- Amenorrhea

- Breast tenderness

- Low back pain

- Mild cramping on one side of the pelvis

- Nausea

- Pain in the lower abdomen or pelvic area

If the area of the abnormal pregnancy ruptures and bleeds, symptoms may get worse. They may include:

- Feeling faint or actually fainting

- Intense pressure in the rectum

- Pain that is felt in the shoulder area

- Severe, sharp, and sudden pain in the lower abdomen

- Internal bleeding due to a rupture may lead to low blood pressure and fainting in around one out of 10 women.

Exams And Tests

The health care provider will do a pelvic exam, which may show tenderness in the pelvic area.

Tests that may be done include:

- Culdocentesis

- Hematocrit

- Pregnancy test

- Quantitative human chorionic gonadotropin (HCG) blood test

- Serum progesterone level

- Transvaginal ultrasound or pregnancy ultrasound

- White blood count

A rise in quantitative HCG levels may help tell a normal (intrauterine) pregnancy from an ectopic pregnancy. Women with high levels should have a vaginal ultrasound to identify a normal pregnancy.

Other tests may be used to confirm the diagnosis, such as:

- Dilatation and curettage (D and C)

- Laparoscopy

- Laparotomy

Treatment

Ectopic pregnancies cannot continue to birth (term). The developing cells must be removed to save the mother's life.

You will need emergency medical help if the area of the ectopic pregnancy breaks open (ruptures). Rupture can lead to shock, an emergency condition. Treatment for shock may include:

- Blood transfusion

- Fluids given through a vein

- Keeping warm

- Oxygen

- Raising the legs

If there is a rupture, surgery (laparotomy) is done to stop blood loss. This surgery is also done to:

- Confirm an ectopic pregnancy

- Remove the abnormal pregnancy

- Repair any tissue damage

In some cases, the doctor may have to remove the fallopian tube.

A minilaparotomy and laparoscopy are the most common surgical treatments for an ectopic pregnancy that has not ruptured. If the doctor does not think a rupture will occur, you may be given a medicine called methotrexate and monitored. You may have blood tests and liver function tests.

Outlook (Prognosis)

One-third of women who have had one ectopic pregnancy are later able to have a baby. A repeated ectopic pregnancy may occur in one-third of women. Some women do not become pregnant again.

The likelihood of a successful pregnancy depends on:

- The woman's age

- Whether she has already had children

- Why the first ectopic pregnancy occurred

> **It's A Fact!**
> The rate of death due to an ectopic pregnancy in the United States has dropped in the last 30 years to less than 0.1%.

Possible Complications

The most common complication is rupture with internal bleeding that leads to shock. Death from rupture is rare.

When To Contact A Medical Professional

If you have symptoms of ectopic pregnancy (especially lower abdominal pain or abnormal vaginal bleeding), call your health care provider. You can have an ectopic pregnancy if you are able to get pregnant (fertile) and are sexually active, even if you use birth control.

Prevention

Most forms of ectopic pregnancy that occur outside the fallopian tubes are probably not preventable. However, a tubal pregnancy (the most common type of ectopic pregnancy) may be prevented in some cases by avoiding conditions that might scar the fallopian tubes.

The following may reduce your risk:

- Avoiding risk factors for pelvic inflammatory disease (PID) such as having many sexual partners, having sex without a condom, and getting sexually transmitted diseases (STDs)
- Early diagnosis and treatment of STDs
- Early diagnosis and treatment of salpingitis and PID
- Stopping smoking

Alternative Names

Tubal pregnancy; Cervical pregnancy; Abdominal pregnancy

Chapter 41

Miscarriage And Stillbirth

Miscarriage

A miscarriage, sometimes called pregnancy loss, is the loss of pregnancy from natural causes before the 20th week of pregnancy. Most miscarriages occur very early in the pregnancy, often before a woman even knows she is pregnant.

Causes

There are many different causes for a miscarriage, some known and others unknown. In most cases, there is nothing a woman can do to prevent a miscarriage.

There are some factors that may contribute to miscarriage:

- The most common cause of miscarriage in the first trimester is a chromosomal abnormality in the fetus. This usually results from a problem with the sperm or egg that prevents the fetus from developing properly.

- During the second trimester, problems with the uterus or cervix can contribute to miscarriage.

- Women with a disorder called polycystic ovary syndrome are three times more likely to miscarry during the early months of pregnancy than women who don't have the syndrome.

About This Chapter: Information in this chapter is from the following publications of the National Institute of Child Health and Human Development (NICHD): "Miscarriage," May 2007; and "Stillbirth," September 2006.

> ## It's A Fact!
> Women who have miscarriages can and often do become pregnant again, with normal pregnancy outcomes.
>
> Source: From "Miscarriage," NICHD, May 2007.

Symptoms And Treatments

Signs of a miscarriage can include:

- Vaginal spotting or bleeding

- Cramping or abdominal pain

- Fluid or tissue passing from the vagina

Although vaginal bleeding is a common symptom when a woman has a miscarriage, many pregnant women have spotting early in their pregnancy but do not miscarry. But, pregnant women who have symptoms such as bleeding should contact their health care provider immediately.

Women who miscarry early in their pregnancy usually do not need any treatment. In some cases, a woman may need a procedure called a dilatation and curettage (D and C) to remove tissue remaining in the uterus. A D and C can be done in a health care provider's office, an outpatient clinic, or a hospital.

Stillbirth

A stillbirth is the loss of pregnancy due to natural causes after the 20th week of pregnancy. It can occur before delivery or during delivery.

Signs

In some cases of stillbirth, the mother may notice a decrease in the movement or kicking of the fetus. In these cases, the health care provider uses an ultrasound, a machine that uses sound waves to create a picture of the fetus, to learn more about its health.

If the fetus has died, an autopsy and placental examination is performed to get information on why the baby died. But it is not always possible to tell why the baby died.

Causes

Causes of a stillbirth may include the following:

- Problems with the placenta, such as an abruption in which the placenta peels away from the uterine wall

- Chromosomal abnormalities resulting from defects in the sperm or egg that make the fetus unable to develop properly

- Other physical problems in the fetus

- Fetuses that are small for their gestational age or not growing at an appropriate rate

- Bacterial infections that can cause complications and death to the fetus

In at least half of all cases, researchers can find no cause for the pregnancy loss.

Medical Procedures For Stillbirth

In some cases it is medically necessary for a woman to deliver the fetus immediately after the diagnosis of a stillbirth.

In other cases, the couple can decide when they want to deliver the fetus.

A health care provider can induce labor or perform a caesarean section to deliver the fetus. A woman will usually go into labor on her own within two weeks after the fetal death.

Quick Tip

If you are pregnant and have concerns about stillbirth, ask your health care provider if there are ways he or she wants you to track movement.

Source: From "Stillbirth," NICHD, September 2006.

Part Five
Childbirth

Chapter 42

Your Developing Baby

First Trimester (Week 1–Week 12)

4 Weeks

At four weeks, your baby has developed in the following ways:

- Your baby's brain and spinal cord have begun to form.

- The heart begins to form.

- Arm and leg buds appear.

- Your baby is now an embryo and one twenty-fifth inch long.

8 Weeks

At eight weeks, your baby has developed in the following ways:

- All major organs and external body structures have begun to form.

- Your baby's heart beats with a regular rhythm.

- The arms and legs grow longer, and fingers and toes have begun to form.

- The sex organs begin to form.

- The eyes have moved forward on the face and eyelids have formed.

- The umbilical cord is clearly visible.

About This Chapter: Information in this chapter is from "Stages of Pregnancy," a publication of the Office on Women's Health, U.S. Department of Health and Human Services, September 2010.

> ## It's A Fact!
> At the end of eight weeks, your baby is a fetus and looks more like a human. Your baby is nearly one inch long and weighs less than one-eighth ounce.

12 Weeks

At 12 weeks, your baby has developed in the following ways:

- The nerves and muscles begin to work together. Your baby can make a fist.

- The external sex organs show if your baby is a boy or girl. A woman who has an ultrasound in the second trimester or later might be able to find out the baby's sex.

- Eyelids close to protect the developing eyes. They will not open again until the 28th week.

- Head growth has slowed, and your baby is much longer. Now, at about three inches long, your baby weighs almost an ounce.

Second Trimester (Week 13–Week 28)

16 Weeks

At 16 weeks, your baby has developed in the following ways:

- Muscle tissue and bone continue to form, creating a more complete skeleton.

- Skin begins to form. You can nearly see through it.

- Meconium develops in your baby's intestinal tract. This will be your baby's first bowel movement.

- Your baby makes sucking motions with the mouth (sucking reflex).

- Your baby reaches a length of about four to five inches and weighs almost three ounces.

20 Weeks

At 20 weeks, your baby has developed in the following ways:

- Your baby is more active. You might feel slight fluttering.

- Your baby is covered by fine, downy hair called lanugo and a waxy coating called vernix. This protects the forming skin underneath.

- Eyebrows, eyelashes, fingernails, and toenails have formed. Your baby can even scratch itself.

- Your baby can hear and swallow.

- Now halfway through your pregnancy, your baby is about six inches long and weighs about nine ounces.

24 Weeks

At 24 weeks, your baby has developed in the following ways:

- Bone marrow begins to make blood cells.

- Taste buds form on your baby's tongue.

- Footprints and fingerprints have formed.

- Real hair begins to grow on your baby's head.

- The lungs are formed, but do not work.

- The hand and startle reflex develop.

- Your baby sleeps and wakes regularly.

- If your baby is a boy, his testicles begin to move from the abdomen into the scrotum. If your baby is a girl, her uterus and ovaries are in place, and a lifetime supply of eggs have formed in the ovaries.

It's A Fact!

At 24 weeks, your baby stores fat and has gained quite a bit of weight. Now at about 12 inches long, your baby weighs about one and a half pounds.

Third Trimester (Week 29–Week 40)

32 Weeks

At 32 weeks, your baby has developed in the following ways:

- Your baby's bones are fully formed, but still soft.

- Your baby's kicks and jabs are forceful.

- The eyes can open and close and sense changes in light.

- Lungs are not fully formed, but practice breathing movements occur.

- Your baby's body begins to store vital minerals, such as iron and calcium.

- Lanugo begins to fall off.

- Your baby is gaining weight quickly, about one-half pound a week. Now, your baby is about 15 to 17 inches long and weighs about four to four and a half pounds.

36 Weeks

At 36 weeks, your baby has developed in the following ways:

- The protective waxy coating called vernix gets thicker.

- Body fat increases. Your baby is getting bigger and bigger and has less space to move around. Movements are less forceful, but you will feel stretches and wiggles.

- Your baby is about 16 to 19 inches long and weighs about six to six and a half pounds.

Weeks 37–40

Between weeks 37 and 40, your baby has developed in the following ways:

- By the end of 37 weeks, your baby is considered full term. Your baby's organs are ready to function on their own.

- As you near your due date, your baby may turn into a head-down position for birth. Most babies present head down.

- At birth, your baby may weigh somewhere between six pounds two ounces and nine pounds two ounces and be 19 to 21 inches long. Most full-term babies fall within these ranges. But healthy babies come in many different sizes.

Chapter 43

Items Your Baby Will Need

Many expectant parents enjoy putting together their baby's layette. This is the clothing and supplies your baby will need in the months ahead. There are countless baby items, and every gadget comes in different shapes, sizes, and brands. So, it can be hard to know what items you will really need or use.

The list in this chapter will give you some ideas about what you might need and want. Ask mothers you know about what items they couldn't live without and brands they liked. Also, keep in mind that the cost of brand-new baby gear can add up. Many new parents keep costs down by borrowing clothes and gear or shopping at consignment stores.

Safety is also an important factor when shopping for supplies. Some products may pose a risk to your baby if safety guidelines are not followed. And used products are more likely than new items to be dangerous.

What Your Baby Will Need At The Hospital

At the hospital, your baby will need the following:

- Undershirt

- An outfit such as a stretch suit, nightgown, or sweater set

- A pair of socks or booties

- Receiving blanket, cap, and heavier blanket or bunting, if the weather is cold

About This Chapter: Information in this chapter is from "Baby's Layette," a publication of the Office on Women's Health, U.S. Department of Health and Human Services, September 2010.

- Diapers and wipes (some hospitals provide an initial supply of these)

- Infant car seat

Quick Tip

If you are overwhelmed by the number of baby products out there, just remember this: Your baby really only needs food, shelter, and you.

Things You'll Need To Transport Your Baby

You will need the following things to transport your baby:

- **Rear-Facing Infant Car Seat:** A proper car seat is the best way to protect your baby on the road and the only legal way to transport your baby in a car. Buying a new seat is best, so that you can be sure the seat is safe and in good condition. Be careful when using an infant car seat outside the car. Do not place a car seat holding a baby on table tops or other elevated surfaces. Improper use of car seats outside the car puts babies at risk of injury and death. Common reasons for car seat-related injuries include falling out of car seats, car seats falling from elevated surfaces, and car seats overturning on soft surfaces.

- **For Walking:** Stroller; soft carrier, sling, or backpack.

- **Diaper Bag:** Since this is something you will be carrying around for about three years, choose one that is comfortable and durable for you.

Items For Your Baby's Room

You will need the following items for your baby's room:

- **Crib And Crib Linens:** Most brand new cribs and mattresses purchased in the United States are safe. If you are planning to use a used crib, make sure it conforms to the current government safety standards. Do not use infant sleep positioners, which are dangerous and not needed.

It's A Fact!

Most hospitals will not discharge the baby unless the car seat is checked for safety and correct installation.

- **Other Furniture:** Changing table; dresser; glider or rocking chair; clothes hamper
- **For Play And Travel:** Play pen or portable crib
- **Smaller Items:** baby monitor; night light/soft lighting

Infant Care Items

You will need the following items to care for your baby:

- Diapers or cloth diapers (test different brands and choose your favorite)
- Receiving blankets
- Clothing
- Breast pump (if you plan to breastfeed)
- Bottles (Be sure to get the correct size of nipples, such as preemie, or newborn.)
- Rectal or digital ear thermometer
- Bathtub
- Washcloths and baby wipes
- Diaper rash ointment and/or petroleum jelly
- Hooded towels
- Diaper disposal system (Good to have, but not necessary.)
- Burp cloths and waterproof lap pads
- Bulb syringe, for suctioning baby's nasal passages if necessary. Your baby's doctor will tell you if, when, and how to do this.
- Baby nail clippers/scissors manicure set

Things You'll Need As Your Baby Gets Older

As your baby gets older, you will need the following items:

- Outlet covers, cabinet locks, and other items to childproof your home
- Toys
- Books
- High chair
- Gates

Chapter 44

Making Your Home Safe For Baby

Your baby is on the way, and there is a lot to think about. Besides making sure that you have baby furniture and clothing for your new son or daughter, you'll want to check that your home is safe. These tips can help you cover all the safety bases.

Before you bring baby home, do the following:

- **Check the safety of your baby's crib and other baby items.** Many new parents welcome hand-me-down baby items from family and friends. Although it's wise to save money, some products could be unsafe if recalled or if parts are missing or loose. Unsafe cribs and other items can put your baby's life in danger. Most brand new cribs and mattresses purchased in the United States are safe. Make sure the crib conforms to the current government safety standards. Also, check to see if hand-me-down items, such as bassinets or portable cribs, have been recalled. Check for recalls and get information on buying a safe crib and mattress at the U.S. Consumer Product Information Safety Commission website.

- **Remove pillows, blankets, and stuffed animals from the crib to prevent your baby from suffocation.**

- **Check to see that smoke detectors and carbon monoxide detectors in your home are working.** Place at least one smoke detector on each level of your home and in halls outside of bedrooms. Have an escape plan in case of fire.

- **Put emergency numbers, including poison control, near each phone.** Have at least one phone in your home connected by land line. Cordless phones do not work when the power is out, and cell phone batteries can run out.

About This Chapter: Information in this chapter is from "Making Your Home Safe For Baby," a publication of the Office on Women's Health, U.S. Department of Health and Human Services, September 2010.

- **Make sure your home or apartment number is easy to see so fire or rescue can locate you quickly in an emergency.**

- **Make sure handrails are installed and secure in stairways.** Always hold the handrail when using stairs, especially when holding your baby.

Your baby will be crawling before you know it. Thinking ahead to the toddler years will help you to take care of other hazards before your baby grows and finds them first. Crawling on your hands and knees will reveal many dangers to your baby. Here are some things to do before your baby is crawling:

- Cover all unused electrical sockets with outlet plugs.

- Keep cords out of baby's reach. Tack up cords to vertical blinds and move furniture, lamps, or electronics to hide cords.

> **It's A Fact!**
> Most babies begin crawling around six to nine months.

- Secure furniture and electronics, such as bookcases and TVs, so they cannot be pulled down on top of your baby.

- Use protective padding to cover sharp edges and corners, such as from a coffee table or fireplace hearth.

- Install safety gates at the bottom and top of stairwells or to block entry to unsafe rooms.

- Use safety latches on cabinets and doors.

- Store all medicines, cleaning products, and other poisons out of baby's reach.

- Remove rubber tips from doorstops or replace with one-piece doorstops.

- Look for and remove all small objects. Objects that easily can pass through the center of a toilet paper roll might cause choking.

- Keep houseplants out of baby's reach. Some plants can poison your baby or make your baby sick.

- Set your water heater temperature to no higher than 125 degrees Fahrenheit. Water that is hotter can cause bad burns.

- Closely supervise your baby around a family pet. Pets need time to adjust to a new baby.

Chapter 45

Taking Classes To Prepare For Baby

CPR—Infant

Cardiopulmonary resuscitation (CPR) is a lifesaving procedure that is performed when an infant's breathing or heartbeat has stopped, as in cases of drowning, suffocation, choking, or injuries. CPR is a combination of:

- Rescue breathing, which provides oxygen to the infant's lungs.
- Chest compressions, which keep the infant's blood circulating.

Permanent brain damage or death can occur within minutes if an infant's blood flow stops. Therefore, you must continue these procedures until the infant's heartbeat and breathing return, or trained medical help arrives.

Considerations

CPR can be lifesaving, but it is best performed by those who have been trained in an accredited CPR course. The procedures described here are not a substitute for CPR training.

All parents and those who take care of children should learn infant and child CPR if they haven't already. This jewel of knowledge is something no parent should be without. (See www .americanheart.org for classes near you.)

Time is very important when dealing with an unconscious infant who is not breathing. Permanent brain damage begins after only four minutes without oxygen, and death can occur as soon as four to six minutes later.

About This Chapter: This chapter begins with information from "CPR—infant," © 2011 A.D.A.M., Inc. Reprinted with permission. Text under the heading "Other Classes" is from "Birthing, Breastfeeding, and Parenting Classes," a publication of the U.S. Department of Health and Human Services, September 2010.

Causes

In infants, major reasons that heartbeat and breathing stop include:

- Choking

- Drowning

- Electrical shock

- Excessive bleeding

- Head trauma or serious injury

- Lung disease

- Poisoning

- Suffocation

Symptoms

- No breathing

- No pulse

- Unconsciousness

First Aid

The following steps are based on instructions from the American Heart Association.

1. Check for responsiveness. Shake or tap the infant gently. See if the infant moves or makes a noise. Shout, "Are you OK?"

2. If there is no response, shout for help. Send someone to call 911. Do not leave the infant yourself to call 911 until you have performed CPR for about two minutes.

3. Carefully place the infant on his or her back. If there is a chance the infant has a spinal injury, two people should move the infant to prevent the head and neck from twisting.

4. Open the airway. Lift up the chin with one hand. At the same time, tilt the head by pushing down on the forehead with the other hand.

5. Look, listen, and feel for breathing. Place your ear close to the infant's mouth and nose. Watch for chest movement. Feel for breath on your cheek.

6. If the infant is not breathing:

- Cover the infant's mouth and nose tightly with your mouth.

- Alternatively, cover just the nose. Hold the mouth shut.

- Keep the chin lifted and head tilted.

- Give two rescue breaths. Each breath should take about a second and make the chest rise.

7. Perform chest compressions:

   - Place two fingers on the breastbone—just below the nipples. Make sure not to press at the very end of the breastbone.

   - Keep your other hand on the infant's forehead, keeping the head tilted back.

   - Press down on the infant's chest so that it compresses about ⅓ to ½ the depth of the chest.

   - Give 30 chest compressions. Each time, let the chest rise completely. These compressions should be FAST and hard with no pausing. Count the 30 compressions quickly: "1,2,3,4, 5,6,7,8,9,10,11,12,13,14,15,16,17,18,19,20,21,22,23,24,25,26,27,28,29,30, off."

8. Give the infant two more breaths. The chest should rise.

9. Continue CPR (30 chest compressions followed by two breaths, then repeat) for about two minutes.

10. After about two minutes of CPR, if the infant still does not have normal breathing, coughing, or any movement, leave the infant if you are alone and call 911.

11. Repeat rescue breathing and chest compressions until the infant recovers or help arrives.

If the infant starts breathing again, place him or her in the recovery position. Periodically re-check for breathing until help arrives.

Do Not

- Lift the infant's chin while tilting the head back to move the tongue away from the windpipe. If a spinal injury is suspected, pull the jaw forward without moving the head or neck. Don't let the mouth close.

- If the infant has signs of normal breathing, coughing, or movement, DO NOT begin chest compressions. Doing so may cause the heart to stop beating.

- Unless you are a health professional, DO NOT check for a pulse. Only a health care professional is properly trained to check for a pulse.

When To Contact A Medical Professional

- If you have help, tell one person to call 911 while another person begins CPR.

- If you are alone, shout loudly for help and begin CPR. After doing CPR for about two minutes, if no help has arrived, call 911. You may carry the infant with you to the nearest phone (unless you suspect spinal injury).

Prevention

Unlike adults, who often require CPR because of a heart attack, most children need CPR because of a preventable accident.

Never underestimate what an infant can do. Play it safe and assume the child is more mobile and more dexterous than you thought possible. Never leave an infant unattended on a bed, table, or other surface from which the infant could roll. Always use safety straps on high chairs and strollers. Never leave an infant in a mesh playpen with one side down. Follow the guidelines for using infant car seats.

Quick Tip

Start teaching your infant the meaning of "Don't touch." The earliest safety lesson is "No!"

Source: © 2011 A.D.A.M., Inc.

Choose age-appropriate toys. Do not give infants toys that are heavy or fragile. Inspect toys for small or loose parts, sharp edges, points, loose batteries, and other hazards.

Create a safe environment and supervise children carefully, particularly around water and near furniture. Keep toxic chemicals and cleaning solutions safely stored in childproof cabinets. Dangers such as electrical outlets, stove tops, and medicine cabinets are attractive to infants and small children.

To reduce the risk of choking accidents, make sure infants and small children cannot reach buttons, watch batteries, popcorn, coins, grapes, or nuts. It is also important to sit with an infant while he or she eats. Do not allow an infant to crawl around while eating or drinking from a bottle.

Never tie pacifiers, jewelry, chains, bracelets, or anything else around an infant's neck or wrists.

Alternative Names

Rescue breathing and chest compressions—infant; Resuscitation—cardiopulmonary—infant; Cardiopulmonary resuscitation—infant

Other Classes

First-time mothers-to-be often have lots of questions and even some worries: How will I know I'm in labor? Will it hurt? Will my baby know how to breastfeed? How do I care for a newborn? Classes to prepare you for childbirth, breastfeeding, infant care, and parenting are great ways to lessen anxiety and build confidence. In some cities, classes might be offered in different languages.

Birthing Classes

Birthing classes often are offered through local hospitals and birthing centers. Some classes follow a specific method, such as Lamaze or the Bradley method. Others review labor techniques from a variety of methods. You might want to read about the different methods beforehand to see if one appeals more to you than others. That way, you will know what to sign up for if more than one type of birthing class if offered. Try to sign up for a class several months before your due date. Classes sometimes fill up quickly. Also, make sure the instructor is qualified.

Most women attend the class with the person who will provide support during labor, such as a spouse, sister, or good friend. This person is sometimes called the labor coach. During class, the instructor will go over the signs of labor and review the stages of labor. She will talk about positioning for labor and birth, and ways to control pain. She also will give you strategies to work through labor pains and to help you stay relaxed and in control. You will practice many of these strategies in class, so you are ready when the big day arrives. Many classes also provide a tour of the birthing facility.

Breastfeeding Classes

Like any new skill, breastfeeding takes knowledge and practice to be successful. Pregnant women who learn about how to breastfeed are more likely to be successful than those who do not. Breastfeeding classes offer pregnant women and their partners the chance to prepare and ask questions before the baby's arrival. Classes may be offered through hospitals, breastfeeding support programs, La Leche League, or local lactation consultants. Ask your doctor for help finding a breastfeeding class in your area.

> ## It's A Fact!
>
> Some hospitals and birthing centers offer sibling classes for soon-to-be brothers and sisters. These classes often help small children get ready for a new baby using fun games and activities.
>
> Source: U.S. Department of Health and Human Services, September 2010.

Parenting Classes

Many first-time parents have never cared for a newborn. Hospitals, community education centers, and places of worship sometimes offer baby care classes. These classes cover the basics, such as diapering, feeding, and bathing your newborn. You also will learn these basic skills in the hospital before you are discharged.

In some communities parenting classes are available. Children don't come with how-to manuals. So some parents appreciate learning about the different stages of child development, as well as practical skills for dealing with common issues, such as discipline or parent-child power struggles. Counselors and social workers often teach this type of class. If you are interested in parenting programs, ask your child's doctor for help finding a class in your area.

Chapter 46

Creating Your Birth Plan

The birth of your baby is one of the most memorable, life-changing, exciting experiences of your life. You will want to spend some time thinking through your hopes and wishes for this special day. Starting with a journal, try to write down as many of your thoughts and plans for your birth as you can. Your journal will help you prioritize and articulate your ideas for creating your birth plan.

A birth plan is a simple, clear, one-page statement of your preferences for the birth of your baby. Having a copy for every person involved in the birth will help each person understand each other and work out communication issues before the big day. Because there are so many aspects of birth to consider, it is best not to wait until the last minute to create your plan. You will want to discuss it with those who will support and care for you.

Try to remember to be flexible, because deviations may be necessary. You will also want to remember the goal: the safe birth of your little bundle of joy. Keeping the goal in mind, the following step-by-step guide will help you create your birth plan.

Compile Considerations

Find out ALL the routine policies and procedures for "mommy care" in your birth setting. If you do not agree with something that is a routine part of birth at your particular setting, you may want to talk further with your health care provider. As you learn about the typical care provided, you will realize areas you want to mention in your plan.

You may want to consider one page for an uncomplicated birth/postpartum and a second page about how to handle complications should they occur. The following list of questions may seem overwhelming, but now is the time to think them through. If a question does not pertain to you, cross it off the list, then prioritize the ones that mean the most to you.

- Who do you want to be there?

- Do you want a doula?

- Will there be children/siblings present?

- Do you want mobility or do you wish to be confined to a bed?

- What activities or positions do you plan to use? (walking, standing, squatting, hands and knees)

- Would you prefer a certain position to give birth?

- What will you do for pain relief? (massage, hot and cold packs, positions, labor imagery, relaxation, breathing exercises, tub or Jacuzzi, medication)

- How do you feel about fetal monitoring?

- How do you plan to keep hydrated? (sips of drinks, ice chips, IV)

- Do you want pain medications, or do you want to avoid them? Do you have preferences for which pain medications you want?

- Would you like an episiotomy? Or, are there certain measures you want to use to avoid one?

- What are your preferences for your baby's care? (when to feed, where to sleep)

- Do you want a routine IV, a heparin/saline block, or nothing at all?

- Do you want to wear your own clothing?

- Do you want to listen to music and have focal points?

- Do you want to use the tub or shower?

- For home and birth center births, what are your plans in case of hospital transport?

- If you need a cesarean, do you have any special requests?

Consult Health Care Provider

Most of the time, health care providers have a set routine of how things are done. They have been trained, and they want what is best for the birth as well. They may or may not be welcoming of your birth plan. They might feel it is a list of demands, or that you may be setting yourself up for failure and disappointment if everything doesn't go precisely as planned.

Keeping in mind that every birth is different and that a "normal" birth may have a wide range of definitions, use wording like "birth preferences," "our wishes for childbirth," "as long as birth progresses normally," or "unless there is an emergency."

After this step, you will feel more confident about your birth plan and have greater confidence in your choice of birth location.

Quick Tip

Make an appointment with the labor and birth area of your hospital or birthing center to have staff look over your plan and provide feedback and suggestions. Kindly request to spend time in an empty birthing or labor room to get a feel for where you will be and what you might want to add to your packing list, like extra pillows, pictures, music.

Confidence And Control

During childbirth, many women feel like they are losing control. A birth plan helps you to feel confident and in control as much as possible and helps you feel part of the decision making even if unexpected events occur.

Try to plan for the unexpected by using phrases like, "If a cesarean becomes necessary..." During birth, if you feel pressured to comply with something you are unsure of, ask if this is an emergency situation; ask if you can have more information on any alternatives and time to think about it. See if they can check back with you in a little while.

The Power Of Positive Thinking

Try to have your birth plan focus on the positive, instead of a list of what you don't want. Use words like, "We hope to" or "We plan to" or "We anticipate." Try not to use phrases like, "We don't want" or "We want to avoid."

Chapter 47

Birthing Centers And Hospital Maternity Services

You'll make plenty of decisions during pregnancy, and choosing where to give birth—whether in a hospital or in a birth center setting—is one of the most important.

Hospitals

Many women fear that a hospital setting will be cold and clinical, but that's not necessarily true. A hospital setting can accommodate a variety of birth experiences.

Traditional hospital births (in which the mother-to-be moves from a labor room to a delivery room and then, after the birth, to a semiprivate room) are still the most common option. Doctors manage the delivery with their patients. In many cases, women in labor are not allowed to eat or drink (possibly due to anesthesia or for other medical reasons), and they may be required to deliver in a certain position.

Pain medications are available during labor and delivery (if the woman chooses); labor may be induced, if necessary; and the fetus is usually electronically monitored throughout the labor. A birth plan can help a woman communicate her preferences about these issues, and doctors will abide by these as much as possible.

In response to a push for more natural birth events, many hospitals now offer more modern options for low-risk births, often known as family-centered care. These may include private rooms with baths (birthing suites) where women can labor, deliver, and recover in one place without having to be moved.

Although a doctor and medical staff are still present, the rooms are usually set up to create a nurturing environment, with warm, soothing colors and features that try to simulate a home-like atmosphere that can be very comforting for new moms. Rooming in—when the baby stays with the mother most of the time instead of in the infant nursery—also may be available.

In addition, many hospitals offer a variety of childbirth and prenatal education classes to prepare parents for the birth experience and parenting classes after birth.

The number of people allowed to attend the birth varies from hospital to hospital. In more traditional settings, as many as three support people are permitted to be with the mother during a vaginal birth. In a family-centered approach, more family members, friends, and sometimes even kids may be allowed. During a routine or nonemergency c-section, usually just one support person is allowed.

If you decide to give birth in a hospital, you will encounter a variety of health professionals:

Obstetrician/gynecologists (OB/GYNs) are doctors with at least four additional years of training after medical school in women's health and reproduction, including both surgical and medical care. They can handle complicated pregnancies and also perform c-sections.

Look for obstetricians who are board-certified, meaning they have passed an examination by the American Board of Obstetrics and Gynecology (ACOG). Board-certified obstetricians who go on to receive further training in high-risk pregnancies are called maternal-fetal specialists or perinatologists.

If you deliver in a hospital, you also might be able to use a certified nurse-midwife (CNM). CNMs are registered nurses who have a graduate degree in midwifery, meaning they're trained to handle normal, low-risk pregnancies and deliveries. Most CNMs deliver babies in hospitals or birth centers, although some do home births.

In addition to obstetricians and CNMs, registered nurses (RNs) attend births to take care of the mother and baby. If you give birth in a teaching hospital, medical students or residents might be present during the birth. Some family doctors also offer prenatal care and deliver babies.

While you're in the hospital, if you choose or if it's necessary for you to receive anesthesia, it will be administered by a trained anesthesiologist. A variety of pain-control measures, including pain medication and local, epidural, and general anesthesia, are available in the hospital setting.

Birth Centers

Women who experience delivery in a birth center are usually those who have already given birth without any problems and whose current pregnancies are considered low risk (meaning they are in good health and are the least likely to develop complications).

Women who are giving birth to multiples, have certain medical conditions (such as gestational diabetes or high blood pressure), or whose baby is in the breech position are considered higher risk and should not deliver in a birth center. Women are carefully screened early in pregnancy and given prenatal care at the birth center to monitor their health throughout their pregnancy.

Natural childbirth is the focus in a birth center. Since epidural anesthesia usually isn't offered, women are free to move around in labor, get in the positions most comfortable to them, spend time in the jacuzzi, etc. The baby is monitored frequently in labor typically with a hand-held Doppler. Comfort measures such as hydrotherapy, massage, warm and cold compresses, and visualization and relaxation techniques are often used. The woman is free to eat and drink as she chooses.

A variety of health care professionals operate in the birth center setting. A birth center may employ registered nurses, CNMs, and doulas (professionally trained providers of labor support and/or postpartum care). Although a doctor is seldom present and medical interventions are rarely done, birth centers may work with a variety of obstetric and pediatric consultants. The professionals affiliated with a birth center work closely together as a team, with the nurse-midwives present and the OB/GYN consultants available if a woman develops a complication during pregnancy or labor that puts her into a higher risk category.

Birth centers do have medical equipment available, including intravenous (IV) lines and fluids, oxygen for the mother and the infant, infant resuscitators, infant warmers, local anesthesia to repair tears and episiotomies (although these are seldom performed), and oxytocin to control postpartum bleeding.

It's A Fact!

A birth center can provide natural pain control and pain control with mild narcotic medications, but if a woman decides she wants an epidural, or if complications develop, she must be taken to a hospital.

Birth centers often provide a homey birth experience for the mother, baby, and extended family. In most cases, birth centers are freestanding buildings, although they may be attached to a hospital. Birth centers may be located in residential areas and generally include amenities such as private rooms with soft lighting, showers, and whirlpool tubs. A kitchen may be available for the family to use.

Look for a birth center that is accredited by the Commission for the Accreditation of Birth Centers (CABC). Some states regulate birth centers, so find out if the birth center you choose has all the proper credentials.

Which One Is Right for You?

How do you decide whether a hospital or a birth center is the right choice for you? If you've chosen a particular health care provider, he or she may only practice at a particular hospital or birth center, so you should discuss your decision. You should also verify your choice with your health insurance carrier to make sure it's covered. In many cases, accredited birth centers as well as hospitals are covered by major insurance companies.

It's A Fact!
If you have any conditions that would classify your pregnancy as higher risk (such as being older than 35, carrying multiple fetuses, or having gestational diabetes or high blood pressure, to name a few), your health care provider may advise you to have your child in a hospital where you and your baby can receive the required medical treatment, if necessary. In fact, you may be ineligible to deliver in a birth center because of your risk factors.

If you desire interventions such as an epidural or continuous fetal monitoring, a hospital is probably the better choice for you.

For a woman without significant problems in her medical history and whose pregnancy has been classified as low risk, a birth center might be an option. Someone who desires a natural birth with minimal medical intervention or pain control may feel more comfortable in a birth center. Because the number of labor and support people you can choose to be present is less limited, if you want to have your entire family participate in the birthing experience, you might consider a birth center.

Once you've decided on either a hospital or a birth center, you may still have to choose which hospital or which birth center. Before you make a choice, you'll have to verify if your health care provider, whether he or she is a doctor or a CNM, will only deliver at certain facilities. In addition, try to get a tour of the hospital or birth center so you can determine for yourself if the staff is friendly and the atmosphere is one in which you'll feel relaxed.

Choosing A Hospital: Questions To Ask

Before your labor pains start, get answers to the following questions.

- Is the hospital easy to get to?

- How is it equipped to handle emergencies?

- What level nursery is available? (Nurseries are rated I, II, or III—a level III neonatal intensive care unit [NICU] is equipped to handle any neonatal emergency. A lower rating may require transportation to a level III NICU.)

- How many deliveries take place at the hospital each year? (A higher number means the hospital has more experience with various birth scenarios.)

- What is the nurse-to-patient ratio? (A ratio of 1:2 is considered good during low-risk labor; a 1:1 ratio is best in complicated cases or during the pushing stage.)

- What are the hospital's statistics for cesarean sections, episiotomies, and mortality? (Keep in mind, though, that these numbers include high-risk and complicated deliveries.)

- How many labor and support people may be present for the birth?

- What procedures are followed after your baby's birth? Can you breastfeed immediately if desired? Is rooming in available?

- How long is the typical postpartum stay for vaginal deliveries? For c-sections?

- Can the baby and the father stay with you in your room around the clock, if you desire?

Choosing A Birth Center: Questions To Ask

- Is the birth center accredited by the Commission for the Accreditation of Birth Centers?

- Is the birth center easy to get to?

- What situations during labor would lead to a transfer to a hospital? How are transfers handled? What emergencies are the transfer facilities able to handle?

- What professionals (such as midwives, doctors, and nurses) are available on staff? On a consulting basis? Are they licensed?

- What childbirth and prenatal education classes are offered?

- What are the center's statistics for hospital transfers, episiotomies, and mortality?

- What procedures are followed after your baby's birth? How long is the typical post-partum stay and how will your baby be examined?

- It's wise to choose where to deliver your baby as early in your pregnancy as possible. That way, if complications do arise, you'll be well informed and can concentrate on your health and the health of your baby.

Chapter 48

Labor And Birth

Spot The Signs Of Labor

As you approach your due date, you will be looking for any little sign that labor is about to start. You might notice that your baby has dropped or moved lower into your pelvis. If you have a pelvic exam during your prenatal visit, your doctor might report changes in your cervix that you cannot feel, but that suggest your body is getting ready.

Some signs suggest that labor will begin very soon. Call your doctor or midwife if you have any of the following signs of labor. Call your doctor even if it's weeks before your due date—you might be going into preterm labor. Your doctor or midwife can decide if it's time to go to the hospital or if you should be seen at the office first.

- You have contractions that become stronger at regular and increasingly shorter intervals.

- You have lower back pain and cramping that does not go away.

- Your water breaks (can be a large gush or a continuous trickle).

- You have a bloody (brownish or red-tinged) mucus discharge. This is probably the mucus plug that blocks the cervix. Losing your mucus plug usually means your cervix is dilating (opening up) and becoming thinner and softer (effacing). Labor could start right away or may still be days away.

About This Chapter: Information in this chapter is from "Labor and birth," a publication of the Office on Women's Health, U.S. Department of Health and Human Services, September 2010.

> **It's A Fact!**
> It's not always easy to know if your water has broken. If your water breaks, it could be a gush or a slow trickle of amniotic fluid. Rupture of membranes is the medical term for your water breaking. Let your doctor know the time your water breaks and any color or odor. Also, call your doctor if you think your water broke, but are not sure. An easy test can tell your doctor if the leaking fluid is urine (many pregnant women leak urine) or amniotic fluid. Often a woman will go into labor soon after her water breaks. When this doesn't happen, her doctor may want to induce (bring about) labor. This is because once your water breaks your risk of getting an infection goes up as labor is delayed.

False Labor

Many women, especially first-time mothers-to-be, think they are in labor when they're not. This is called false labor. Practice contractions called Braxton Hicks contractions are common in the last weeks of pregnancy or earlier. The tightening of your uterus might startle you. Some might even be painful or take your breath away. So, how can you tell if your contractions are true labor?

Use a watch or clock to keep track of the time one contraction starts to the time the next contraction starts, as well as how long each contraction lasts. With true labor, contractions become regular, stronger, and more frequent. Braxton Hicks contractions are not in a regular pattern, and they taper off and go away. Some women find that a change in activity, such as walking or lying down, makes Braxton Hicks contractions go away. This won't happen with true labor. Even with these guidelines, it can be hard to tell if labor is real. If you ever are unsure if contractions are true labor, call your doctor.

Stages Of Labor

Labor occurs in three stages. When regular contractions begin, the baby moves down into the pelvis as the cervix both effaces (thins) and dilates (opens). How labor progresses and how long it lasts are different for every woman. But each stage features some milestones that are true for every woman.

> **It's A Fact!**
> Most babies' heads enter the pelvis facing to one side, and then rotate to face down.

First Stage

The first stage begins with the onset of labor and ends when the cervix is fully opened. It is the longest stage of labor, usually lasting about 12 to 19 hours. Many women spend the early part of this first stage at home. While at home, time your contractions and keep your doctor up to date on your progress. Your doctor will tell you when to go to the hospital or birthing center.

At the hospital, your doctor will monitor the progress of your labor by periodically checking your cervix, as well as the baby's position and station (location in the birth canal). As you near the end of the first stage of labor, contractions become longer, stronger, and closer together. Many of the positioning and relaxation tips you learned in childbirth class can help now.

Sometimes, medicines and other methods are used to help speed up labor that is progressing slowly. Many doctors will rupture the membranes. Although this practice is widely used, studies show that doing so during labor does not help shorten the length of labor.

Your doctor might want to use an electronic fetal monitor to see if blood supply to your baby is okay. For most women, this involves putting two straps around the mother's abdomen. One strap measures the strength and frequency of your contractions. The other strap records how the baby's heartbeat reacts to the contraction.

The most difficult phase of this first stage is the transition. Contractions are very powerful, with very little time to relax in between, as the cervix stretches the last, few centimeters. Many women feel shaky or nauseated. The cervix is fully dilated when it reaches 10 centimeters.

Second Stage

The second stage involves pushing and delivery of your baby. It usually lasts 20 minutes to two hours. You will push hard during contractions, and rest between contractions. Pushing is hard work, and a support person can really help keep you focused.

When the top of your baby's head fully appears (crowning), your doctor will tell you when to push and deliver your baby. Your doctor may make a small cut, called an episiotomy, to enlarge the vaginal opening. Most women in childbirth do not need an episiotomy. Sometimes, forceps (a tool shaped like salad tongs) or suction is used to help guide the baby through the birth canal.

Third Stage

The third stage involves delivery of the placenta (afterbirth). It is the shortest stage, lasting five to 30 minutes. Contractions will begin five to 30 minutes after birth, signaling that it's time to deliver the placenta. You might have chills or shakiness. Labor is over once the placenta is delivered. Your doctor will repair the episiotomy and any tears you might have. Now, you can rest and enjoy your newborn.

It's A Fact!

Most babies present head down. If a baby's feet or buttocks are in position to deliver first, the baby is said to be breech. Breech deliveries increase the risk that the baby will suffer health problems or die. If your baby is breech, your doctor may try to turn the baby a few weeks before your due date simply by pushing your abdomen. Your doctor may also suggest a cesarean delivery.

Managing Labor Pain

Some women do fine with natural methods of pain relief alone. Many women blend natural methods with medications that relieve pain.

Natural Methods Of Pain Relief

Many natural methods help women to relax and make pain more manageable. Things women do to ease the pain include: trying breathing and relaxation techniques; taking warm showers or baths; getting massages; using heat and cold, such as heat on lower back and cold washcloth on forehead; having the supportive care of a loved one, nurse, or doula; finding comfortable positions while in labor (stand, crouch, sit, walk, etc.); using a labor ball; listening to music.

Medical Methods Of Pain Relief

While you're in labor, your doctor, midwife, or nurse should ask if you need pain relief. It is her job to help you decide what option is best for you. Nowadays women in labor have many pain relief options that work well and pose small risks when given by a trained and experienced doctor. Doctors also can use different methods for pain relief at different stages of labor. Still, not all options are available at every hospital and birthing center. Plus your health history, allergies, and any problems with your pregnancy will make some methods better than others.

Most medicines used to manage pain during labor pass freely into the placenta. Ask your doctor how pain relief methods might affect your baby or your ability to breastfeed after delivery.

Inducing Labor

Sometimes, a doctor or midwife might need to induce (bring about) labor. The decision to induce labor often is made when a woman is past her due date but labor has not yet begun or when there is concern about the baby or mother's health.

It's A Fact!

The doctor or midwife can use medicines and other methods to open a pregnant woman's cervix, stimulate contractions, and prepare for vaginal birth.

Elective labor induction has become more common in recent years. This is when labor is induced at term but for no medical reason. Some doctors may suggest elective induction due to a woman's discomfort, scheduling issues, or concern that waiting may lead to complications. If your doctor suggests inducing labor, talk to your doctor about the possible harms and benefits for both mother and baby, such as the risk of c-section and the risk of low birthweight.

Cesarean Birth

Cesarean delivery, also called c-section, is surgery to deliver a baby. The baby is taken out through the mother's abdomen. Most cesarean births result in healthy babies and mothers. But c-section is major surgery and carries risks. Healing also takes longer than with vaginal birth.

Reasons For C-Sections

Your doctor might recommend a c-section if she or he thinks it is safer for you or your baby than vaginal birth. Some c-sections are planned. But most c-sections are done when unexpected problems happen during delivery. Even so, there are risks of delivering by c-section. Limited studies show that the benefits of having a c-section may outweigh the risks when one or more of the following conditions are true:

Quick Tip

Public health experts think that many c-sections are unnecessary. So it is important for pregnant women to get the facts about c-sections before they deliver. Women should find out what c-sections are, why they are performed, and the pros and cons of this surgery.

- The mother is carrying more than one baby (twins, triplets, etc.)

- The mother has health problems including human immunodeficiency virus (HIV) infection, herpes infection, and heart disease

- The mother has dangerously high blood pressure

- The mother has problems with the shape of her pelvis

- There are problems with the placenta

- There are problems with the umbilical cord

- There are problems with the position of the baby, such as breech

- The baby shows signs of distress, such as a slowed heart rate

- The mother has had a previous c-section

Chapter 49

Recovering From Birth

New mothers must take special care of their bodies after giving birth and while breastfeeding. Doing so will help you to regain your energy and strength. When you take care of yourself, you are able to best care for and enjoy your baby.

Getting Rest

The first few days at home after having your baby are a time for rest and recovery—physically and emotionally. You need to focus your energy on yourself and on getting to know your new baby. Even though you may be very excited and have requests for lots of visits from family and friends, try to limit visitors and get as much rest as possible. Don't expect to keep your house perfect. You may find that all you can do is eat, sleep, and care for your baby. And that is perfectly okay. Learn to pace yourself from the first day that you arrive back home. Try to lie down or nap while the baby naps. Don't try to do too much around the house. Allow others to help you and don't be afraid to ask for help with cleaning, laundry, meals, or with caring for the baby.

Physical Changes

After the birth of your baby, your doctor will talk with you about things you will experience as your body starts to recover.

- You will have vaginal discharge called lochia. It is the tissue and blood that lined your uterus during pregnancy. It is heavy and bright red at first, becoming lighter in flow and color until it goes away after a few weeks.

About This Chapter: Information in this chapter is from "Recovering from birth," a publication of the Office on Women's Health, U.S. Department of Health and Human Services, September 2010.

- You might also have swelling in your legs and feet. You can reduce swelling by keeping your feet elevated when possible.

- You might feel constipated. Try to drink plenty of water and eat fresh fruits and vegetables.

- Menstrual-like cramping is common, especially if you are breastfeeding. Your breast milk will come in within three to six days after your delivery. Even if you are not breastfeeding, you can have milk leaking from your nipples, and your breasts might feel full, tender, or uncomfortable.

- Follow your doctor's instructions on how much activity, like climbing stairs or walking, you can do for the next few weeks.

Your doctor will check your recovery at your postpartum visit, about six weeks after birth. Ask about resuming normal activities, as well as eating and fitness plans to help you return to a healthy weight. Also ask your doctor about having sex and birth control. Your period could return in six to eight weeks, or sooner if you do not breastfeed. If you breastfeed, your period might not resume for many months. Still, using reliable birth control is the best way to prevent pregnancy until you want to have another baby.

Some women develop thyroid problems in the first year after giving birth. This is called postpartum thyroiditis. It often begins with overactive thyroid, which lasts two to four months. Most women then develop symptoms of an underactive thyroid, which can last up to a year. Thyroid problems are easy to overlook as many symptoms, such as fatigue, sleep problems, low energy, and changes in weight, are common after having a baby. Talk to your doctor if you have symptoms that do not go away. An underactive thyroid needs to be treated. In most cases, thyroid function returns to normal as the thyroid heals. But some women develop permanent underactive thyroid disease, called Hashimoto's disease, and need lifelong treatment.

Regaining A Healthy Weight And Shape

Both pregnancy and labor can affect a woman's body. After giving birth you will lose about 10 pounds right away and a little more as body fluid levels decrease. Don't expect or try to lose additional pregnancy weight right away. Gradual weight loss over several months is the safest way, especially if you are breastfeeding. Nursing mothers can safely lose a moderate amount of weight without affecting their milk supply or their babies' growth.

A healthy eating plan along with regular physical fitness might be all you need to return to a healthy weight. If you are not losing weight or losing weight too slowly, cut back on foods with added sugars and fats, like soft drinks, desserts, fried foods, fatty meats, and alcohol. Keep in mind, nursing mothers should avoid alcohol. By cutting back on extras, you can focus on healthy, well-balanced food choices that will keep your energy level up and help you get the nutrients you and your baby need for good health. Make sure to talk to your doctor before you start any type of diet or exercise plan.

Quick Tip

The U.S. Department of Agriculture's (USDA's) online, interactive tool can help you choose foods based on your baby's nursing habits and your energy needs. Visit http://www.mypyramid.gov/mypyramidmoms/pyramidmoms_plan.aspx to figure out how much you need to eat, choose healthy foods, and get the vitamins and minerals you need.

Feeling Blue

After childbirth you may feel sad, weepy, and overwhelmed for a few days. Many new mothers have the baby blues after giving birth. Changing hormones, anxiety about caring for the baby, and lack of sleep all affect your emotions.

Be patient with yourself. These feelings are normal and usually go away quickly. But if sadness lasts more than two weeks, go see your doctor. Don't wait until your postpartum visit to do so. You might have a serious but treatable condition called postpartum depression. Postpartum depression can happen any time within the first year after birth.

Signs of postpartum depression include the following:

- Feeling restless or irritable
- Feeling sad, depressed, or crying a lot
- Having no energy
- Having headaches, chest pains, heart palpitations (the heart being fast and feeling like it is skipping beats), numbness, or hyperventilation (fast and shallow breathing)
- Not being able to sleep, being very tired, or both
- Not being able to eat and weight loss
- Overeating and weight gain
- Trouble focusing, remembering, or making decisions

- Being overly worried about the baby

- Not having any interest in the baby

- Feeling worthless and guilty

- Having no interest or getting no pleasure from activities like sex and socializing

- Thoughts of harming your baby or yourself

Some women don't tell anyone about their symptoms because they feel embarrassed or guilty about having these feelings at a time when they think they should be happy. Don't let this happen to you. Postpartum depression can make it hard to take care of your baby. Infants with mothers who have postpartum depression can have delays in learning how to talk. They can have problems with emotional bonding. Your doctor can help you feel better and get back to enjoying your new baby. Therapy and/or medicine can treat postpartum depression.

Emerging research suggests that one in 10 new fathers may experience depression during or after pregnancy. Although more research is needed, having depression may make it harder to be a good father and perhaps affect the baby's development. Having depression may also be related to a mother's depression. Expecting or new fathers with emotional problems or symptoms of depression should talk to their doctors. Depression is a treatable illness.

Quick Tip

Call 911 or your doctor if you have thoughts of harming yourself or your baby.

Part Six
Your Newborn

Chapter 50

Your Baby's First Hours Of Life

After months of waiting, finally, your new baby has arrived. Mothers-to-be often spend so much time in anticipation of labor, they don't think about or even know what to expect during the first hours after delivery. Read on so you will be ready to bond with your new bundle of joy.

What Newborns Look Like

You might be surprised by how your newborn looks at birth. If you had a vaginal delivery, your baby entered this world through a narrow and boney passage. It's not uncommon for newborns to be born bluish, bruised, and with a misshapen head. An ear might be folded over. Your baby may have a complete head of hair or be bald. Your baby also will have a thick, pasty, whitish coating, which protected the skin in the womb. This will wash away during the first bathing.

Once your baby is placed into your arms, your gaze will go right to his or her eyes. Most newborns open their eyes soon after birth. Eyes will be brown or bluish-gray at first. Looking over your baby, you might notice that the face is a little puffy. You might notice small white bumps inside your baby's mouth or on his or her tongue. Your baby might be very wrinkly. Some babies, especially those born early, are covered in soft, fine hair, which will come off in a couple of weeks. Your baby's skin might have various colored marks, blotches, or rashes, and fingernails could be long. You might also notice that your baby's breasts and penis or vulva are a bit swollen.

How your baby looks will change from day to day, and many of the early marks of childbirth go away with time. If you have any concerns about something you see, talk to your doctor. After a few weeks, your newborn will look more and more like the baby you pictured in your dreams.

About This Chapter: Information in this chapter is from "Your baby's first hours of life," a publication of the Office on Women's Health, U.S. Department of Health and Human Services, September 2010.

Bonding With Your Baby

Spending time with your baby in those first hours of life is very special. Although you might be tired, your newborn could be quite alert after birth. Cuddle your baby skin-to-skin. Let your baby get to know your voice and study your face. Your baby can see up to about two feet away. You might notice that your baby throws his or her arms out if someone turns on a light or makes a sudden noise. This is called the startle response. Babies also are born with grasp and sucking reflexes. Put your finger in your baby's palm and watch how she or he knows to squeeze it. Feed your baby when she or he shows signs of hunger.

Medical Care For Your Newborn

Right after birth babies need many important tests and procedures to ensure their health. Some of these are even required by law. But as long as the baby is healthy, everything but the Apgar test can wait for at least an hour. Delaying further medical care will preserve the precious first moments of life for you, your partner, and the baby. A baby who has not been poked and prodded may be more willing to nurse and cuddle. So before delivery, talk to your doctor or midwife about delaying shots, medicine, and tests. At the same time, please don't assume everything is being taken care of. As a parent, it's your job to make sure your newborn gets all the necessary and appropriate vaccines and tests in a timely manner.

The following tests and procedures are recommended or required in most hospitals in the United States.

Apgar Evaluation

The Apgar test is a quick way for doctors to figure out if the baby is healthy or needs extra medical care. Apgar tests are usually done twice: one minute after birth and again five minutes after birth. Doctors and nurses measure five signs of the baby's condition:

- Heart rate
- Breathing
- Activity and muscle tone
- Reflexes
- Skin color

Apgar scores range from zero to 10. A baby who scores seven or more is considered very healthy. But a lower score doesn't always mean there is something wrong. Perfectly healthy babies often have low Apgar scores in the first minute of life.

It's A Fact!

In more than 98 percent of cases, the Apgar score reaches seven after five minutes of life. When it does not, the baby needs medical care and close monitoring.

Eye Care

Your baby may receive eye drops or ointment to prevent eye infections he or she can get during delivery. Sexually transmitted infections (STIs), including gonorrhea and chlamydia, are a main cause of newborn eye infections. These infections can cause blindness if not treated.

Medicines used can sting and/or blur the baby's vision. So you may want to postpone this treatment for a little while.

Some parents question whether this treatment is really necessary. Many women at low risk for STIs do not want their newborns to receive eye medicine. But there is no evidence to suggest that this medicine harms the baby.

It is important to note that even pregnant women who test negative for STIs may get an infection by the time of delivery. Plus, most women with gonorrhea and/or chlamydia don't know it because they have no symptoms.

Vitamin K Shot

The American Academy of Pediatrics recommends that all newborns receive a shot of vitamin K in the upper leg. Newborns usually have low levels of vitamin K in their bodies. This vitamin is needed for the blood to clot. Low levels of vitamin K can cause a rare but serious bleeding problem. Research shows that vitamin K shots prevent dangerous bleeding in newborns.

Newborns probably feel pain when the shot is given. But afterwards babies don't seem to have any discomfort. Since it may be uncomfortable for the baby, you may want to postpone this shot for a little while.

Newborn Metabolic Screening

Doctors or nurses prick your baby's heel to take a tiny sample of blood. They use this blood to test for many diseases. All babies should be tested because a few babies may look healthy but have a rare health problem. A blood test is the only way to find out about these problems. If found right away, serious problems like developmental disabilities, organ damage, blindness, and even death might be prevented.

All 50 states and U.S. territories screen newborns for phenylketonuria (PKU), hypothyroidism, galactosemia, and sickle cell disease. But many states routinely test for up to 30 different diseases. The March of Dimes recommends that all newborns be tested for at least 29 diseases.

Quick Tip

You can find out what tests are offered in your state by contacting your state's health department or newborn screening program. Or, you can contact the National Newborn Screening and Genetics Resource Center.

Hearing Test

Most babies have a hearing screening soon after birth, usually before they leave the hospital. Tiny earphones or microphones are used to see how the baby reacts to sounds. All newborns need a hearing screening because hearing defects are not uncommon and hearing loss can be hard to detect in babies and young children. When problems are found early, children can get the services they need at an early age. This might prevent delays in speech, language, and thinking. Ask your hospital or your baby's doctor about newborn hearing screening.

Hepatitis B Vaccine

All newborns should get a vaccine to protect against the hepatitis B virus (HBV) before leaving the hospital. Sadly, one in five babies at risk of HBV infection leaves the hospital without receiving the vaccine and treatment shown to protect newborns, even if exposed to HBV at birth. HBV can cause a lifelong infection, serious liver damage, and even death.

The hepatitis B vaccine (HepB) is a series of three different shots. The American Academy of Pediatrics and the Centers for Disease Control (CDC) recommend that all newborns get the first HepB shot before leaving the hospital. If the mother has HBV, her baby should also get a hepatitis B immune globulin (HBIG) shot within 12 hours of birth. The second HepB shot should be given one to two months after birth. The third HepB shot should be given no earlier than 24 weeks of age, but before 18 months of age.

Complete Checkup

Soon after delivery most doctors or nurses also do the following:

- Measure the newborn's weight, length, and head.

- Take the baby's temperature.

- Measure the baby's breathing and heart rate.

- Give the baby a bath and clean the umbilical cord stump.

Chapter 51

Breastfeeding

Why Breastfeeding Is Important

Breastfeeding Protects Babies

1. **Early breast milk is liquid gold.** Known as liquid gold, colostrum is the thick yellow first breast milk that you make during pregnancy and just after birth. This milk is very rich in nutrients and antibodies to protect your baby. Although your baby only gets a small amount of colostrum at each feeding, it matches the amount his or her tiny stomach can hold.

2. **Your breast milk changes as your baby grows.** Colostrum changes into what is called mature milk. By the third to fifth day after birth, this mature breast milk has just the right amount of fat, sugar, water, and protein to help your baby continue to grow. It is a thinner type of milk than colostrum, but it provides all of the nutrients and antibodies your baby needs.

3. **Breast milk is easier to digest.** For most babies—especially premature babies—breast milk is easier to digest than formula. The proteins in formula are made from cow's milk, and it takes time for babies' stomachs to adjust to digesting them.

4. **Breast milk fights disease.** The cells, hormones, and antibodies in breast milk protect babies from illness. This protection is unique; formula cannot match the chemical make-up of human breast milk. In fact, among formula-fed babies, ear infections and diarrhea are more common. Formula-fed babies also have higher risks of other diseases, including the following:

About This Chapter: Information in this chapter is from "Your Guide to Breastfeeding," a publication of the Office on Women's Health, U.S. Department of Health and Human Services, January 2011.

- Necrotizing enterocolitis, a disease that affects the gastrointestinal tract in preterm infants.

- Lower respiratory infections

- Atopic dermatitis, a type of skin rash

- Asthma

- Obesity

- Type 1 and type 2 diabetes

- Childhood leukemia

Breastfeeding has also been shown to lower the risk of SIDS (sudden infant death syndrome).

It's A Fact!

Formula feeding can raise health risks in babies, but there are rare cases in which formula may be a necessary alternative. Very rarely, babies are born unable to tolerate milk of any kind. These babies must have soy formula. Formula may also be needed if the mother has certain health conditions and she does not have access to donor breast milk.

Mothers Benefit From Breastfeeding

1. **Breastfeeding can make your life easier.** Breastfeeding may take a little more effort than formula feeding at first. But it can make life easier once you and your baby settle into a good routine. When you breastfeed, there are no bottles and nipples to sterilize. You do not have to buy, measure, and mix formula. And there are no bottles to warm in the middle of the night.

2. **Breastfeeding can save money.** Formula and feeding supplies can cost well over $1,500 each year, depending on how much your baby eats. Breastfed babies are also sick less often, which can lower health care costs.

3. **Breastfeeding can feel great.** Physical contact is important to newborns. It can help them feel more secure, warm, and comforted. Mothers can benefit from this closeness, as well. Breastfeeding requires a mother to take some quiet relaxed time to bond. The skin-to-skin contact can boost the mother's oxytocin levels. Oxytocin is a hormone that helps milk flow and can calm the mother.

4. Breastfeeding can be good for the mother's health, too. Breastfeeding is linked to a lower risk of these health problems in women:

- Type 2 diabetes

- Breast cancer

- Ovarian cancer

- Postpartum depression

Experts are still looking at the effects of breastfeeding on osteoporosis and weight loss after birth. Many studies have reported greater weight loss for breastfeeding mothers than for those who don't. But more research is needed to understand if a strong link exists.

5. Nursing mothers miss less work. Breastfeeding mothers miss fewer days from work because their infants are sick less often.

Breastfeeding Benefits Society

The nation benefits overall when mothers breastfeed. Recent research shows that if 90 percent of families breastfed exclusively for six months, nearly 1,000 deaths among infants could be prevented. The United States would also save $13 billion per year—medical care costs are lower for fully breastfed infants than for never-breastfed infants. Breastfed infants typically need fewer sick care visits, prescriptions, and hospitalizations.

Breastfeeding also contributes to a more productive workforce because mothers miss less work to care for sick infants. Employer medical costs are also lower.

Breastfeeding is also better for the environment. There is less trash and plastic waste compared to that produced by formula cans and bottle supplies.

Breastfeeding During An Emergency

When an emergency occurs, breastfeeding can save lives:

- Breastfeeding protects babies from the risks of a contaminated water supply.
- Breastfeeding can help protect against respiratory illnesses and diarrhea. These diseases can be fatal in populations displaced by disaster.
- Breast milk is the right temperature for babies and helps to prevent hypothermia when the body temperature drops too low.
- Breast milk is readily available without needing other supplies.

Finding Support And Information

While breastfeeding is natural, you still may need some advice. There are many sources of support available for breastfeeding mothers. You can seek help from different types of health professionals, organizations, and members of your own family. Under the Affordable Care Act (health care reform), more and more women will have access to breastfeeding support without any out-of-pocket costs. And don't forget, friends who have successfully breastfed can be a great source of information and encouragement.

Health Professionals Who Help With Breastfeeding

Pediatricians, obstetricians, and certified nurse-midwives can help you with breastfeeding. Other special breastfeeding professionals include:

- **International Board Certified Lactation Consultant (IBCLC):** Lactation consultants are credentialed breastfeeding professionals with the highest level of knowledge and skill in breastfeeding support. IBCLCs are experienced in helping mothers to breastfeed comfortably by helping with positioning, latch, and a wide range of breastfeeding concerns. Many IBCLCs are also nurses, doctors, speech therapists, dietitians, or other kinds of health professionals. Ask your hospital or birthing center for the name of a lactation consultant who can help you. Or, you can go to http://www.ilca.org to find an IBCLC in your area.

- **Breastfeeding Peer Counselor Or Educator:** A breastfeeding counselor can teach others about the benefits of breastfeeding and help women with basic breastfeeding challenges and questions. A peer means a person has breastfed her own baby and is available to help other mothers. Some breastfeeding educators have letters after their names like CLC (Certified Lactation Counselor) or CBE (Certified Breastfeeding Educator). Educators have special breastfeeding training but not as much as IBCLCs. These professionals still can be quite helpful.

- **Doula:** A doula is professionally trained and experienced in giving social support to birthing families during pregnancy, labor, and birth and at home during the first few days or weeks after birth. Doulas who are trained in breastfeeding can help you be more successful with breastfeeding after birth.

Mother-To-Mother Support

Other breastfeeding mothers can be a great source of support. Mothers can share tips and offer one another encouragement. There are many ways you can connect with other breastfeeding mothers:

- Ask your health care provider or hospital staff to recommend a support group.

- Search your phone book or the internet for a breastfeeding center near you. These centers may offer support groups.

- Find a local La Leche League support group by visiting the organization's website at http://www.llli.org/.

- Search the internet for breastfeeding message boards and chats. (These resources can be great for sharing tips, but do not rely on websites for medical advice—talk to your health care provider.)

WIC Program

Food, nutrition counseling, and access to health services are provided to low-income women, infants, and children under the Special Supplemental Nutrition Program for Women, Infants, and Children. This program is popularly known as WIC (women, infants, and children). Breastfeeding mothers supported by WIC may receive educational materials, peer counselor support, an enhanced food package, breast pumps, and other supplies.

Breastfeeding mothers are also eligible to participate in WIC longer than nonbreastfeeding mothers. To find contact information for your local WIC program, visit http://www.fns.usda.gov/wic/Breastfeeding/breastfeedingmainpage.htm or call the national office at 703-305-2746.

The National Breastfeeding Helpline

The National Breastfeeding Helpline from the Office on Women's Health has trained breastfeeding peer counselors to provide support by phone. The counselors can help answer common breastfeeding questions. They can also help you decide if you need to see a doctor or lactation consultant. The Helpline is available for all breastfeeding mothers, partners, prospective parents, family members, and health professionals seeking to learn more about breastfeeding. The Helpline is open from Monday through Friday, from 9 a.m. to 6 p.m., EST. If you call after hours, you will be able to leave a message, and a breastfeeding peer counselor will return your call on the next business day. Help is available in English or Spanish. Call 800-994-9662 for support.

Quick Tip

Learn more about breastfeeding basics and find other online resources at http://www.womenshealth.gov/ breastfeeding.

Before You Give Birth

To prepare for breastfeeding, the most important thing you can do is have confidence in yourself. Committing to breastfeeding starts with the belief that you can do it. Other steps you can take to prepare for breastfeeding include the following:

1. Get good prenatal care, which can help you avoid early delivery. Babies born too early often need special care, which can make breastfeeding harder.

2. Take a breastfeeding class.

3. Ask your health care provider to recommend a lactation consultant. You can establish a relationship before the baby comes, or be ready if you need help after the baby is born.

4. Talk to your health care provider about your health. Discuss any breast surgery or injury you may have had. If you have depression or are taking medications, discuss treatment options that can work with breastfeeding.

5. Tell your health care provider that you would like to breastfeed your newborn baby as soon as possible after delivery. The sucking instinct is very strong within the first hour of life.

6. Talk to friends who have breastfed or consider joining a breastfeeding support group.

Talk To Fathers, Partners, And Other Family Members About How They Can Help

Breastfeeding is more than a way to feed a baby—it becomes a lifestyle. And fathers, partners, and other special support persons can be involved in the breastfeeding experience, too. Partners and family members can:

- Support the breastfeeding relationship by being kind and encouraging.

- Show their love and appreciation for all of the work that is put into breastfeeding.

- Be good listeners when a mother needs to talk through breastfeeding concerns.

- Make sure the mother has enough to drink and gets enough rest, help around the house, and help caring for other children at home.

- Give emotional nourishment to the child through playing and cuddling.

It's A Fact!

Fathers, partners, and other people in the mother's support system can benefit from breastfeeding, too. Not only are there no bottles to prepare, but many people feel warmth, love, and relaxation just from sitting next to a mother and baby during breastfeeding.

Chapter 52

Bringing Your Baby Home

Whether your baby comes home from the hospital right away, arrives later (perhaps after a stay in the neonatal intensive care unit), or comes through an adoption agency, the homecoming of your little one is a major event you've probably often imagined. Here's how to be prepared.

Leaving The Hospital

Moms-to-be sometimes pack clothes for the trip home before even going to the hospital—or they may wait to see what the weather brings and have their partner bring clothing for both themselves and the baby. Plan to bring loose-fitting clothing for yourself with a drawstring or elastic waist because you most likely won't fit into your pre-pregnancy outfits yet.

Babies are frequently overdressed for the first trip home. In warm weather, it's practical to dress your baby in a T-shirt and diaper and wrap him or her in a baby blanket. Hats aren't necessary, but they can be a cute finishing touch, especially for the first picture in the hospital.

If it's cold, add a snowsuit and an extra blanket. Chances are much better that you'll bring home a calm, contented baby if you don't spend a lot of time at the hospital trying to dress your newborn in a complicated outfit that requires pushing and pulling your baby's arms and legs.

If you haven't already made the arrangements with your baby's health care provider, make sure to ask when the baby's first checkup should be scheduled before you leave the hospital. Depending on the circumstances, some premature babies also go home with a special monitor for checking breathing and heart rate, and you may be taught infant cardiopulmonary resuscitation (CPR).

About This Chapter: Information in this chapter is from "Bringing Your Baby Home," April 2011, reprinted with permission from www.kidshealth.org. Copyright © 2011 The Nemours Foundation. This information was provided by KidsHealth, one of the largest resources online for medically reviewed health information written for parents, kids, and teens. For more articles like this one, visit www.KidsHealth.org, or www.TeensHealth.org.

But whether your baby is full-term or premature, don't feel rushed out the door—have your questions answered before you leave the hospital. And if you find yourself wondering about anything—from bathing to breastfeeding to burping—ask your nurse, lactation consultant, or your baby's doctor.

The Car Trip

The most important item for the trip home is a proper child safety seat (car seat). Every state requires parents to have one before leaving the hospital because it's one of the best ways to protect your baby.

Even for a short trip, it's never safe for one of you to hold your baby in your arms while the other drives. Your baby could be pulled from your arms and thrown against the dashboard by a quick stop.

Consider buying, renting, or borrowing a car seat before your baby's born, when you have time to choose carefully. There are two kinds of car seats for babies: infant-only seats (which must be replaced when your baby weighs 22 to 35 pounds, depending on the type of seat) and convertible seats that accommodate both infants and older children.

Infant-only seats are designed for rear-facing use only and fit infants better than convertible seats. The American Academy of Pediatrics (AAP) recommends that infants and toddlers ride in a rear-facing seat until they are two years old or until they have reached the maximum weight and height limits recommended by the manufacturer. (If your baby exceeds the weight recommended by the manufacturer before the second birthday, you'll need to use a convertible seat designed for bigger babies.)

Some parents of newborns find that a "travel system" (which includes a stroller and an infant-only car seat that can be attached to the stroller) makes it much smoother to transition babies—especially sleeping ones—from the car to the stroller.

Convertible seats face toward the rear until your baby is at least two years old or has reached the maximum weight and height limits recommended by the manufacturer. A child who reaches the height and weight limits before age two is safest in a bigger convertible seat and kept rear facing. Kids who are small can remain in rear-facing seats even after age two. (Follow the manufacturer's guidelines for when to turn the seat.)

Never put a rear-facing infant or convertible seat in the front seat of your car—always use the rear seat. Passenger-side airbags in the front seat cabin are hazardous for both rear- and forward-facing car seats, and most accidents happen at the front passenger area of the car. When it's cold, strap your baby in snugly first, then put blankets over the baby.

If you borrow a car seat, make sure that it's not more than six years old and was never in a crash (even if it looks OK, it could be structurally unsound). Avoid seats that are missing parts or aren't labeled with the manufacture date and model number (you'll have no way to know about recalls).

Also, check the seat for the manufacturer's recommended expiration date. If you have any doubts about the seat's history, or if it's cracked or shows signs of wear and tear, don't use it.

When buying a new seat, it's important to remember that there isn't one type of seat that's safest or best; get one that fits and can be correctly installed in your car. And higher price doesn't necessarily indicate a seat's quality—it could simply mean the seat has added features that you may or may not want. Also, be sure to register your new seat so you can be notified of any problems or recalls.

The most common problem involving car seats is improper installation (according to the National Highway Traffic Safety Administration, the majority of all car seats are installed incorrectly). Recently, LATCH (Lower Anchors and Tethers for Children) car seats have become standard in the United States, but a large percentage of these seats are improperly installed too.

Don't trust illustrations or store displays. Follow the manufacturer's instructions (and keep them handy). Ask your doctor or nurse about local resources where your car seat can be checked by someone specifically trained to evaluate car seat installations. Many hospitals, police and fire stations, and even car dealerships offer this type of service for free. Make sure that the evaluation is done by someone trained and experienced.

If you're bringing your baby home from the intensive care unit, bring the car seat to the hospital ahead of time, so the staff can see if it will work for your baby. If special health concerns rule out a standard restraint, ask your child's doctor to recommend car seats for children with special needs.

For more information on the proper use of child safety seats, read the Nemour Foundation's article on auto safety (available at http://kidshealth.org/parent/firstaid_safe/outdoor/auto.html).

Quick Tip

Ask at your prenatal classes, health care provider's office, hospital, and insurance company about rental or loan programs for car seats—they're quite common.

First-Time Feelings

Don't be surprised if you have mixed emotions as you bring your baby home, especially if this is your first child. You'll likely be nervous. In fact, you may actually feel terrified as you realize that you've given up a certain amount of control over your life.

If your baby wasn't with you much at the hospital, you may not know what sort of schedule your little bundle of joy will keep. But you'll know before long—although babies' schedules do change a lot during those early months. You'll be less stressed if you don't overschedule yourself and can go with the flow.

Depending upon your labor and delivery experience, you may feel physically drained and sore. Your hormones may be struggling to catch up, too. Meanwhile, your partner may feel a little left out if you're totally engrossed with the baby.

You might have other kids awaiting the arrival of this newest family member. Or you may be dealing with a pet who's wondering what's suddenly drawn everyone's attention. Frequently, the expectations of new grandparents, competitive siblings, or friends can also make the homecoming stressful.

Your baby's first extended crying period at home will be difficult. Remember: young babies typically cry for one to five hours within a 24-hour period, and can't always be calmed. Crying usually decreases gradually after the first several weeks. Although it may seem impossible now, in a few months it will be difficult to recall your baby's seemingly endless crying episodes.

The Home Front

Introducing your baby to others at home can be challenging. If you have other kids, be sure to spend some quality time with each of them. Some parents bring home gifts from the new baby for big brothers and sisters. At first, you can expect some jealousy, especially if the main focus of your attention for several years suddenly has new competition. Encourage siblings to "help" you care for this newest family member.

If you have a pet, ask your partner to bring home a blanket with the baby's scent on it and place it near the pet—even before leaving the hospital. Then, when you come home, the pet will already be somewhat familiar with the baby. But remember to never leave pets alone with newborns.

Family And Friends

Ask your partner to be the gatekeeper for visitors and to limit the number of guests at first. You'll be glad later on if you take some time now to rest and become comfortable with your new situation. Although babies typically aren't shy around strangers for the first three months or so, they may become overstimulated and tired if too many people are around.

If you have voice mail or a telephone answering machine, consider changing your message to give the vital statistics of your new arrival. You might say something like: "Our newest family member has arrived. Her name is Julia Marie; she was born on Tuesday, and weighed 7 pounds, 10 ounces. We're all fine and adjusting to our new life. If you'd like us to call you back when it's convenient, please leave your name and number."

Quick Tip

Don't be shy about accepting visitors slowly. Ask anyone who's ill to wait until they're feeling well and no longer contagious before they visit. You shouldn't hesitate to ask visitors to wash their hands before holding your baby because a newborn baby's immune system is not fully developed.

When To Call The Doctor

Your baby's health care provider expects calls from new parents on many topics, including breast-feeding and health concerns. They'd rather have you call than worry about something needlessly.

If you wonder whether you should call the doctor's office, do it, especially if you see something unexpected or different that concerns you. Call if you see any of these signs:

- Rectal temperature of 100.4° F (38° C) or higher (in babies younger than two months)
- Symptoms of dehydration (crying without tears, sunken eyes, a depression in the soft spot on baby's head, no wet diapers in six to eight hours)
- A soft spot that bulges when your baby's quiet and upright
- A baby that is difficult to rouse
- Rapid or labored breathing (call 911 if your baby has breathing difficulty and begins turning bluish around the lips or mouth)
- Repeated forceful vomiting or an inability to keep fluids down
- Bloody vomit or stool
- More than eight diarrhea stools in eight hours

If your concern is urgent, call your doctor and take your child to the emergency room. Remember, with young infants, minor conditions can sometimes change quickly.

Chapter 53

Newborn Care And Safety

Bathing An Infant

Bath time can be fun. But you need to be very careful with your child around water. Most drowning deaths in children happen at home, most times when the caregiver leaves a child alone in the bathroom. Do not leave your child alone around water, not even for a few seconds.

Ways To Prevent Bathing Accidents

These tips can help you prevent accidents in the bath:

- Stay close enough to your child so that you can reach out and hold him or her if he or she slips or falls in the tub.

- Use non-skid decals or a mat inside the tub to prevent slipping.

- Use toys in the tub to keep your child busy and sitting down, and away from the faucet.

- Keep the temperature of your water heater below 120° F to prevent burns.

- Keep all sharp objects, such as razors and scissors, out of your child's reach.

- Unplug all electric items, such as hair dryers and radios.

- Empty the tub after bath time is over.

- Keep the floor and your child's feet dry to prevent slipping.

About This Chapter: This chapter begins with Information from "Bathing an Infant," © 2011 A.D.A.M., Inc. Reprinted with permission. "Newborn Care" and "Sudden Infant Death Syndrome (SIDS)" are from "Newborn Care and Safety," Office on Women's Health, U.S. Department of Health and Human Services. The chapter concludes with "When to Call the Baby's Doctor," Office on Women's Health, DHHS, March 2009.

Extra Tips For Newborns

You will need to be extra careful when bathing your newborn:

- Have a towel ready to wrap your newborn in to dry and keep him or her warm right after the bath.
- Keep your baby's umbilical cord dry.
- Use warm, not hot, water. Place your elbow under the water to check temperature.
- Wash your baby's head last so that his or her head does not get too cold.
- Bathe your baby every three days.

Bathroom Safety

Other tips that can protect your child in the bathroom are:

- Store medicines in the child-proof containers they came in. Keep the medicine cabinet locked.
- Keep cleaning products out of reach of children.
- Keep bathroom doors closed so your child cannot get in when they are not being used.
- Place a door knob cover over the outside door handle.
- Do not ever leave your child alone in the bathroom.
- Place a lid lock on the toilet seat to keep a curious toddler from drowning.

Newborn Care

If this is your first baby, you might worry that you are not ready to take care of a newborn. You're not alone. Lots of new parents feel unprepared when it's time to bring their new babies home from the hospital. You can take steps to help yourself get ready for the transition home.

Taking a newborn care class during your pregnancy can prepare you for the real thing. But feeding and diapering a baby doll isn't quite the same. During your hospital stay, make sure to ask the nurses for help with basic baby care. Don't hesitate to ask the nurse to show you how to do something more than once. Remember, practice makes perfect. Before discharge, make sure you—and your partner—are comfortable with these newborn care basics:

- Handling a newborn, including supporting your baby's neck
- Changing your baby's diaper

- Bathing your baby

- Dressing your baby

- Swaddling your baby

- Feeding and burping your baby

- Cleaning the umbilical cord

- Caring for a healing circumcision

- Using a bulb syringe to clear your baby's nasal passages

- Taking a newborn's temperature

- Tips for soothing your baby

Quick Tip

Before leaving the hospital, ask about home visits by a nurse or health care worker. Many new parents appreciate somebody checking in with them and their baby a few days after coming home. If you are breastfeeding, ask whether a lactation consultant can come to your home to provide follow-up support, as well as other resources in your community, such as peer support groups.

Many first-time parents also welcome the help of a family member or friend who has been there. Having a support person stay with you for a few days can give you the confidence to go at it alone in the weeks ahead. Try to arrange this before delivery.

Your baby's first doctor's visit is another good time to ask about any infant care questions you might have. Ask about reasons to call the doctor. Also ask about what vaccines your baby needs and when. Infants and young children need vaccines because the diseases they protect against can strike at an early age and can be very dangerous in childhood. This includes rare diseases and more common ones, such as the flu.

Sudden Infant Death Syndrome (SIDS)

Since 1992, the American Academy of Pediatrics has recommended that infants be placed to sleep on their backs to reduce the risk of sudden infant death syndrome (SIDS), also called crib death. SIDS is the sudden and unexplained death of a baby under one year of age. Even though there is no way to know which babies might die of SIDS, there are some things that you can do to make your baby safer:

- Always place your baby on his or her back to sleep, even for naps. This is the safest sleep position for a healthy baby to reduce the risk of SIDS.

- Place your baby on a firm mattress, such as in a safety-approved crib. For more information on crib safety, contact the Consumer Product Safety Commission. Research has shown that placing a baby to sleep on soft mattresses, sofas, sofa cushions, waterbeds, sheepskins, or other soft surfaces raises the risk of SIDS.

- Remove soft, fluffy, and loose bedding and stuffed toys from your baby's sleep area. Make sure you keep all pillows, quilts, stuffed toys, and other soft items away from your baby's sleep area.

- Do not use infant sleep positioners. Using a positioner to hold an infant on his or her back or side for sleep is dangerous and not needed.

Tummy Time

Many moms know to place newborns on their backs when it's time to sleep. Babies who sleep on their backs are less likely to suffer from sudden infant death syndrome (SIDS). But babies still need to develop their neck, shoulder, and arm muscles. The best way to help your newborn build her muscles is to give her some tummy time while she's awake.

The American Academy of Pediatrics has some great tips for strengthening your baby's muscles. When she's awake, place her on her stomach to see how much she can move on her own. A baby younger than two months old may struggle to raise her head to look around, but may still be able to lift her head for a few seconds.

While your baby is on her stomach, extend her arms and place a rolled-up receiving blanket underneath her chest and arms. Keep your newborn on her belly for a few seconds at a time each day until she can work her way up to holding her head up for longer. You can motivate her by bringing yourself down to her eye level so she can look at you. You can also try placing a rattle or other attractive toy in front of her to get her attention.

These exercises will strengthen your baby's neck and arm muscles, so that when she's around four months old, she'll be able to hold her head and chest up. Once she achieves this milestone, she'll need less head and neck support when you hold her. Her new upper body strength will help her remain steady and upright when she's learning to sit up at around five months of age. She'll also need these skills when she's learning to roll over and crawl.

As with all baby activities, keep a close watch on her and never leave your baby unattended.

Source: From "Tummy time," © 2008 March of Dimes Birth Defects Foundation. All rights reserved. For additional information, contact the March of Dimes at their website www.marchofdimes.com.

- Make sure everyone who cares for your baby knows to place your baby on his or her back to sleep and about the dangers of soft bedding. Talk to child care providers, grandparents, babysitters, and all caregivers about SIDS risk. Remember, every sleep time counts.

- Make sure your baby's face and head stay uncovered during sleep. Keep blankets and other coverings away from your baby's mouth and nose. The best way to do this is to dress the baby in sleep clothing so you will not have to use any other covering over the baby. If you do use a blanket or another covering, make sure that the baby's feet are at the bottom of the crib, the blanket is no higher than the baby's chest, and the blanket is tucked in around the bottom of the crib mattress.

- Do not allow smoking around your baby. Don't smoke before or after the birth of your baby and make sure no one smokes around your baby.

- Don't let your baby get too warm during sleep. Keep your baby warm during sleep, but not too warm. Your baby's room should be at a temperature that is comfortable for an adult. Too many layers of clothing or blankets can overheat your baby.

- Some mothers worry if the baby rolls over during the night. However, by the time your baby is able to roll over by herself, the risk for SIDS is much lower. During the time of greatest risk, two to four months of age, most babies are not able to turn over from their backs to their stomachs.

When To Call The Baby's Doctor

One of the toughest and most nerve-racking things for new moms is figuring out when to call the doctor. As a general rule of thumb, trust your instincts. If you suspect something is not right, you should always call the doctor. Even small changes in eating, sleeping, and crying can be signs of serious problems for newborns.

Call your pediatrician if your baby has any of the following symptoms:

- No urine in first 24 hours at home

- No bowel movement in the first 48 hours at home

- Trouble breathing, very rapid breathing (more than 60 breaths per minute) or blue lips or fingernails

- Pulling in of the ribs when breathing

- Wheezing, grunting, or whistling sounds when breathing

- Rectal temperature above 100.4° F or below 97.8° F

- Persistent cough

- Nosebleeds

- Yellow or greenish mucus in the eyes

- Pus or red skin at the base of the umbilical cord stump

- Yellow color in whites of the eye and/or skin (jaundice) that gets worse three days after birth

- Circumcision problems—worrisome bleeding at the circumcision site, bloodstains on diaper or wound dressing larger than the size of a grape

- Vomiting

- Diarrhea—This can be hard to detect, especially in breastfed newborns. Diarrhea often has a foul smell and can be streaked with blood or mucus. Diarrhea is usually more watery or looser than normal. Any significant increase in the number or appearance of your newborn's regular bowel movements may suggest diarrhea.

- Fewer than six wet diapers in 24 hours

- A sunken soft spot (fontanel) on the baby's head

- Refuses several feedings or eats poorly

- Hard to waken or unusually sleepy

- Extreme floppiness, lethargy, or jitters

- Crying more than usual and very hard to console

Part Seven
Teen Parenting Problems
And Solutions

Chapter 54

Completing Your Education

As a pregnant teenage student or a teenage parent, you have the same right as any other student to continue your education. Also, you are legally required to attend school.

Here are some of your rights:

- You can stay in your current school or program.

- You cannot be excluded from any school program you qualify for, including magnet, honors, or special education, because of pregnancy or parenthood.

- If you are pregnant, you may choose to attend one of the voluntary specialized programs for pregnant students.

- If you are a teenage parent without child care, you may be able to transfer to a high school or educational program with a child care center on campus.

If You Have Dropped Out Of School Or Fear You May Have To Drop Out

You can get help to find a program that will make it easier to return and graduate or one that will help you prepare to take the General Equivalency Diploma (GED) test to get an Equivalency Certificate. It can be slow going, but DON'T give up! Get the help you need to continue your education and to look forward to a better future for yourself, your child, and your family.

About This Chapter: Information in this chapter is excerpted from "Pregnant? A Teen Parent? Protect Your Future: Stay In School!" a publication of Public Counsel, the public interest law firm of the Los Angeles County and Beverly Hills Bar Associations. 2010. © 2010 Public Counsel. All rights reserved. Reprinted with permission. To view the complete text of this booklet, and additional information, visit www.publicounsel.org.

> **Quick Tip**
> You have many choices: get all the information you need to make the best choice.

When you are facing a lot of problems that make it hard to stay in school or go back to school, you can get help to tackle those problems. School staff can help you get connected with a school program that can work for you. If something else stands in the way, they can also give you information about child care resources, counseling, health care, parenting and support groups, and other assistance you may need to stay in school. Talk to a counselor, school nurse or psychologist, the principal, or a teacher at your school. Keep asking questions until you get the help and information you need. They are there to help you!

You Have The Right To Be Treated With Respect By Everyone At School

No one can treat you differently from other students because you are pregnant or because you are a teen parent. School staff cannot treat you differently whether or not you are married. You deserve to be treated with respect whether you have had an abortion, miscarriage, or need to take time off from school for the birth of your baby. School staff may not allow other students to treat you with disrespect.

As A Pregnant Student Or Teen Parent, You Have A Right To Take Part In All School Activities

You can participate in any classes or school-related activities, including physical education (PE), unless your doctor says you need to limit your physical activity. You can be in honors or awards ceremonies, run for student offices, take part in school clubs and after-school activities, attend field trips, and join in all graduation activities.

> **It's A Fact!**
> Something else important to remember: you have legal rights you might not realize you have.

You Have A Right As Well As A Duty To Make Up School Work You Miss When You Have Excused Absences

You will need to provide a note or appointment card to excuse your absence from school if:

- You are absent due to an illness or condition related to your pregnancy and have a note from your doctor or health care provider.

- You or your child has a medical appointment that can only be made during school hours.

- You are absent for the birth of your child or recovery from childbirth.

- You are absent to care for your sick child.

You Are Responsible For Making Up Work You Miss And You Must Be Allowed Opportunities To Do That

When possible, it is better to plan in advance to make up work that you will miss. In any case, making up missed work is a right of any student who is absent from school due to health-related conditions.

You Have A Right To Get The Help, Support, And Information You Need To Continue Your Education

This includes the right to be informed about optional alternative educational programs that may meet your special needs or let you fill in school credits you are missing. Your school counselor, teacher, or principal can help you make progress toward your goal of graduation or earning your GED.

You Have The Right To Have Your Privacy Respected

- Your health and personal information should be kept confidential (private) just as any other student's information is kept private.

- That means any information about your pregnancy, whether you have children, and if you are married or not is private.

- School staff should not discuss your health or other private information with anyone else without your permission. Staff also cannot use this information against you when you ask for letters of recommendation or when you are being considered for educational or job opportunities or scholarships.

- One exception to this rule of privacy is when there is a concern that you or any other student may have been abused or you are a danger to yourself or others. In this situation, school staff will need to make a report to a child protective service agency to get help.

You Have A Right To Expect Your School To Make Reasonable Changes Or Adjustments To Support Your Successful School Participation

Changes to help a pregnant student remain in school might include: a hall pass to use the restroom as needed, being released early from class at lunch or recess to avoid lines and crowds, or being assigned, when possible, to classes that meet on a lower floor or are closer together—especially during later months of pregnancy. Often schools make similar adjustments for students with other medical conditions or physical challenges. You deserve the same support whenever such changes are possible.

Chapter 55

Considering Emancipation From Your Parents

Emancipation

Emancipation means you are legally separated from your parents or guardian, and they no longer have to support you. Some people call this a divorce from the parents and, like any divorce, can bring good or bad feelings between you and your folks.

LEGALLY, emancipation is the process by which youth who are 14 through 17 years of age may become freed from the custody and control of their parents or guardian. If you do become emancipated, you give up the right to be supported financially by your parents. At the same time, you gain the right to make most of your own decisions and control of most BUT NOT ALL aspects of your life.

Changes That Will Happen In Your Life If You Become Emancipated

Emancipation makes important changes in your relationships with parents, guardians, and public agencies:

- You will lose your right to have financial support—your basic living expenses and health care—paid by your parents or guardian.

About This Chapter: Information in this chapter is excerpted from "So You Want to Become Emancipated?" a publication of Public Counsel, the public interest law firm of the Los Angeles County and Beverly Hills Bar Associations, 2010–2011. © 2011 Public Counsel. All rights reserved. Reprinted with permission. To view the complete text of this booklet, and additional information, visit www.publicounsel.org. Although some of the material is specific to California laws and programs, the general principles of emancipation are relevant for any teen considering emancipation.

- Your parents or guardian will no longer be legally or financially responsible for any injuries you cause to others.

- Becoming an emancipated minor does not automatically make you eligible for public benefits.

- You will be given the right to handle your own affairs. For example, you will be able to:

  - Live where you choose

  - Sign binding contracts

  - Keep and spend your own earnings

  - Get a work permit without your parent's consent

  - Sue someone in your own name

  - Consent to all of your own medical, dental, and psychiatric care

  - Stay out as late as you want

  - Sign up for school or college

What Will Not Change For You If You Become Emancipated

There are certain laws that always apply to minors, even after they become emancipated:

- You must go to school. The compulsory education laws require minors to stay in school until they graduate from high school or reach the age of eighteen.

- You cannot work as many hours as you want. You still have to follow all child labor laws and work permit rules.

- Statutory rape laws still apply to you. If you have sex, you or your partner could get in trouble with the law, especially if there is a big age difference or the relationship is abusive (unless you are married to your partner).

- You cannot legally drink alcohol. Even if emancipated, you may not legally drink alcohol until you turn 21.

- You cannot vote. Emancipation does not lower the voting age. You still must be eighteen to vote.

You Don't Need To Be Emancipated To Get Some Kinds Of Health Care

Even if you are living with your parents and are not emancipated, you can get some kinds of health care for free and without anyone telling your parents. This health care program is called "Medi-Cal Minor Consent Services." It covers family planning, birth control, abortion, and pregnancy care, as well as treatment for drug or alcohol problems, mental health problems, sexually transmitted diseases, rape and sexual assault. You can apply for Medi-Cal Minor Consent Services at health clinics, family planning clinics, or county welfare offices.

So, if you are thinking about emancipation just to get health care, you may want to see if you can get the care you need without having to be emancipated.

Qualifying For Emancipation

There are three ways a minor may become emancipated:

1. **If You Are Married:** Marriage for any teen under the age of 18 requires written consent by parents or guardian and a court order.

2. **By Enlisting In The Armed Services:** Both parental and armed services permission are required if you are under 18.

3. **By Going To Court And Having The Judge Declare You Emancipated ("Judicial Declaration"):** To use this method for emancipation, you must first satisfy the following six requirements:

   - You must be at least 14 years of age at the time you begin to seek legal emancipation.

   - You must NOT be living with your parents or legal guardian. The court wants to be sure you have made a living arrangement where you plan to stay indefinitely. In other words, they want to see more than a temporary address. Saying you are staying with a friend is not enough.

   - Your parents or legal guardian must have consented or acquiesced to your living away from them. Parental consent is generally required for a teen to become emancipated. This can be shown in two ways. One way is to get your parents to sign a consent and attach it to the Petition for Emancipation. If your parents sign this form, it may be easier for you to become emancipated. If your parents won't sign this form, you may be able to show the court that your parents have "acquiesced." If you are living away from home and your parents know all about this but they are not strongly objecting or trying to bring you back home to live, a judge MAY interpret their lack of action as "acquiescence" or agreement to your living arrangement.

- You must manage your own financial affairs. The court needs to be sure you have income earned only by you and that you make the decisions on how that income is spent. You will need to show evidence that you pay your own bills, especially for such necessary things as housing, food, and clothing. It is best if you can show that you actually exchange your money for the things you need. Even if you could argue that you trade housework for room and board, it is better if you can arrange to receive money for the work you do and then use that money to pay rent. While there is no set amount a youth must earn, the judge will examine your finances closely to make certain your income meets expenses. Some judges may deny your request to be emancipated if your only source of income is welfare (CalWORKs).

- Your source of income must be legal. This means you must not earn your living from criminal activities.

- The emancipation must be in your best interest. This requirement allows the judge a great deal of freedom in deciding whether to declare you emancipated. Even if you meet the other five requirements, a judge who feels it is not in your best interest to become emancipated can deny your petition. In court, your parents or anyone else may object to your emancipation and try to persuade the judge that it is not in your best interest.

Myths About Emancipation

Automatic Emancipation When A Girl Gives Birth

You might have heard that when a girl gives birth, she is automatically emancipated. This is ABSOLUTELY NOT true. Having a baby does not mean you are automatically emancipated. Any teen under 18 who has a baby must still legally live with her parents or guardian. Also, if you need cash aid, the law says you must live with a parent or relative, or in an adult-supervised program such as a group home.

But this rule does not apply to Medi-Cal or Food Stamps and there are exceptions. For example, if you or your child's health or safety would be at risk if you lived with a parent, or you have already lived apart from your parents for 12 months. If you need cash aid and don't live with a parent or relative, ask the CalWORKs eligibility worker to refer you to a MINOR PARENT SERVICES caseworker to see if you qualify for one of the exceptions.

Forced Emancipation

Parents cannot force you to become emancipated. There are some parents who would like their child to be emancipated because it means the parents are no longer legally responsible for providing financially for their child. However, emancipation is meant to be an improved step in the youth's life, not a way for parents to get out of their responsibilities.

Some Things To Think About Before Emancipation

- Be sure you really can support yourself without financial help from your parents (including health insurance) as emancipation means giving up your rights to parental support.

- When considering emancipation, you should think about worst case scenarios such as job loss or illness that might prevent you from working or taking care of yourself.

- There is a way of undoing emancipation after it has been granted. However, you should think of emancipation as a permanent situation when you are deciding whether or not to file a petition.

- Have you given up on trying to make your relationship with your parents work? Are you willing to risk having a complete break with them, that could be permanent, and perhaps upsetting other family members as well?

- Keep this in mind: All teenagers become "emancipated" on their 18th birthday without filing a petition or going through this process.

- So take your time in making this decision.

It's A Fact!

If you will be 18 in six months or less, there isn't time to complete the court process for emancipation, which takes four to six months.

Chapter 56

Finding A Place To Live

A Place To Live

Where Can My Baby And I Live?

Perhaps you are wondering about things, such as

- whether you may or must keep living in your parent's home

- whether you can get housing on your own

- whether you're eligible for housing assistance from the government

This chapter will help answer your questions.

Living With Your Parents

Can My Parents Make Me Leave Home Because I Am Pregnant Or Have A Child?

If you are a minor child, your parents must provide shelter for you. It is against the law for your parents to "kick you out" so that you have to find your own shelter or sleep outside. This doesn't mean that your parents must let you live in their home, however. They may provide shelter

About This Chapter: *Pregnancy and Parenting: A Legal Guide for Adolescents, Second Edition* (English Version). Reprinted with permission of the University of North Carolina Chapel Hill School of Government, Copyright 2006. This copyrighted material may not be reproduced in whole or in part without the express written permission of the School of Government, CB# 3330 UNC Chapel Hill, Chapel Hill, North Carolina 27599-3330; telephone: 919-966-4119; fax 919-962-2707; Web address: www.sog.unc.edu. This publication was written specifically to help explain North Carolina law, though it may also provide helpful information to others.

for you in their home, or they may arrange for you to stay somewhere else (as long as the place meets basic needs). Examples of places where your parents could arrange for you to stay are

- with a relative or a family friend,

- in a boarding school,

- in a maternity home, or

- in some other place where treatment is provided (such as a hospital or a group home).

It's A Fact!

Your pregnancy or the birth of your child doesn't change your parents' legal duty to care for and supervise you. If they fail to meet this duty, the department of social services (DSS) can ask a court to find that you are neglected. Your parents don't have to house their grandchildren, though. Under the law, as long as you are an unemancipated minor child, you are expected to live where your parent or guardian tells you to live.

What If I Want To Leave My Parent's Home?

Experts believe that, in most cases, it is better for a teen mother to live at home with her parents after her baby is born. This belief is based on studies showing that young mothers who live with their parents are more likely to finish high school (possibly because live-at-home teen mothers receive more encouragement and/or more help with child care).

Because of this belief that home is usually the best place, many laws and funding programs try to encourage young mothers to stay at home. For example, leaving your parent's home may keep you from getting money from the government (Temporary Assistance for Needy Families, or TANF) to help support your child.

Must A Minor Parent Always Live In A Parent's Home To Get Cash Assistance (TANF)?

Not always. There are two exceptions to this rule. You don't have to live at home if

- you are a teen parent who is married or emancipated, or

- living in your parent's home puts your or your child's physical or emotional health at risk.

It's A Fact!

Under federal law, an unmarried parent who is 17 or younger and has custody of a child older than 12 weeks must be in school or involved in another educational activity and must live at home or in an approved, adult-supervised setting in order to receive government assistance.

Where Can I Live Besides My Parent's Home?

Sometimes a minor mother moves out of her parent's home with no plan for where she and her baby will stay. The young mother may then try living with a series of relatives and friends, but this may not be good for her or her child. If you are moving from place to place, it is very hard to stay in school, to find and keep a job, and to keep up with appointments for your child and yourself, including appointments that keep you eligible for benefits such as Medicaid and TANF. It's even hard to keep up with your mail. For those reasons and perhaps more, you need an adult to help you if you have been asked to leave home or have decided to leave on your own and have no place to stay where your needs will be met. (If you are living with a man you're not married to, the department of social services (DSS) will not consider you to be living in an appropriate adult-supervised arrangement.) If you don't know an adult who can help you, try to find one at school, the police or sheriff's department, the health department, the department of social services, a recreation center, or at a church, synagogue, or mosque. Look for places that show the yellow sign that says "Safe Place." The adults in places with these signs will call someone to meet with you and help you make a plan for yourself and your child.

Can My Parents Keep My Child While Making Me Live Elsewhere?

Your parents may not keep your child (their grandchild) while you are forced to live somewhere else, except in the following situations:

Quick Tip

If you can't live at home because physical or emotional harm might come to you or your child, the department of social services (DSS) must help you find a suitable, adult-supervised place to live. If you think you or your child might be at risk in your parent's home, call DSS and ask for the Child Protective Services section. Tell them that you are reporting your situation and ask them to investigate. They must tell you whether they will investigate, and if they do look into your situation, they must tell you what they decide.

- You are in detention, jail, or prison

- You are in a hospital or other treatment place and can't care for the child

- The department of social services and/or court has given them custody of their grand-child (your child)

Renting Your Own Apartment, House, Or Mobile Home (Trailer)

Can I Rent A Place For Myself?

Probably not. Owners and rental agents for apartments, houses, and mobile homes usually will not sign leases with minors. Also, utility companies that provide water, electricity, natural gas, and heating oil usually won't start these services in a minor's name. This is because, under the law, a minor is not responsible for a contract that he or she signs. So, even if you signed a lease for housing, the landlord probably couldn't collect the rent money if you didn't pay. You may have an adult relative or friend who is willing to sign a lease for you so that you can have your own place. If so, the adult is listed as the person renting the apartment, house, or trailer. He or she is the tenant, which makes him or her legally responsible for the rent and for paying for damage to the property. You and your child are listed as occupants. An adult who signed for your apartment, house, or trailer would be taking on a big responsibility, and it's important for you to know that. It's also important for you to understand a few laws and legal definitions about renting a place to live.

What Is A Lease?

A lease is a contract or legally enforceable agreement between a landlord (the owner of the property) and a tenant (the person who is renting the property). In the lease, the landlord and tenant agree on the rules for the rental of the property. Once the landlord and tenant both sign the lease, they are required to do what the lease says (unless the lease says something that is illegal under the landlord–tenant laws). Rental leases can be either written or spoken, depending on how long the landlord and tenant agree the lease will last. It is usually much better to have a lease in writing. That way, everyone is clear about their responsibilities under the lease and many misunderstandings can be avoided.

What Should Be In A Lease?

These are important things you should look for in a lease:

- The address of the property being rented

- The name and address of the landlord

- How much the rent is per week or month

- How much the deposit is and how you can get it back (A deposit is money that a tenant gives a landlord before moving in, which the landlord can use to pay for damage the tenant might do to the housing unit.)

- Exactly when rent must be paid

- How long you are renting for (This is called the "term of the lease"—for example, some leases require the tenant to rent the property for six months or a year, while other leases only call for renting one month at a time.)

- How the tenant and landlord must notify each other about ending the lease

A lease should also make clear whether the tenant or landlord must pay the utility bills and how the property is to be maintained. Some leases also say who—or at least how many people—may live in the house, apartment, or mobile home. The adult who helps you rent a place to live will be violating the lease if the lease names who may live in the house or apartment and you and your child are not named.

What Are A Landlord's And A Tenant's Main Duties?

The tenant (or a responsible adult if the tenant is a minor) must pay the rent and not damage the property. In return, the landlord must keep the property in a reasonable condition. If your community has a minimum housing code (rules about health and safety in housing), then the landlord must follow that code. If the landlord doesn't make necessary repairs after you inform him of the problem and you believe that your health or safety is at risk, you should report the situation to your local housing office. It is illegal for your landlord to take action against you by, for example, increasing the rent or trying to evict you, because you or the person signing the lease reported the poor condition of the property.

Can I Be Put Out Of An Apartment Before The Lease Is Up?

If the rent isn't paid on time, a landlord may try to have a tenant put out (evicted). Some landlords try to use methods that are illegal. A landlord may not try to make you leave by hassling you, locking you out, putting your things in the street, or turning off the electricity, gas, water, or other essential services. Instead, the law says that unless the lease says otherwise, the landlord must notify the tenant to pay the rent or else the rental agreement will be over.

Public Assistance For Housing

Can I Get Public Assistance For Housing?

You may know that some people in your community get government assistance in buying or renting a home, and you may want similar assistance to rent an apartment. Once you're 18 you may be able to get public assistance for housing. However, most public housing authorities have rules that stop you from even getting on a waiting list for an apartment or for rental assistance until your 18th birthday. And even then, you're not guaranteed housing assistance. In the United States, there is no legal right to safe, decent, and affordable housing. Instead, housing assistance is seen as a benefit that the government may provide. In recent years, the federal government has set aside little money for housing assistance. As a result, many public housing agencies have cut back the number of people they serve.

What Should I Do If I'm Homeless?

Many cities and towns have homeless shelters. The law allows minors to use emergency shelters for the homeless without their parents' permission. However, if the shelter staff let you stay, they will contact your parents within a day or so. Some shelters will take a minor mother with her child—but unfortunately, quite a few will not. To find out if there's a shelter where you are, call the police or the department of social services (DSS).

The National Runaway Switchboard (NRS)—1-800-RUNAWAY (1-800-786-2929), http://www.1800runaway.org/—tries to help minors anywhere in the United States who have run away from home (or are thinking about it), or who are homeless for any reason. NRS gets about two thousand calls a year from North Carolina.

The National Runaway Switchboard

- Takes calls from anyone, 24 hours a day, every day of the year
- Keeps calls confidential (NRS doesn't have Caller ID)
- Does not call the police—unless you ask them to
- Is required by law to report suspected abuse, neglect, or dependency to DSS
- Is not connected to any religious organization
- Doesn't judge callers
- Doesn't go out and look for kids
- Gives messages to families

- Will arrange conference calls between a minor and her family

- Refers kids to shelter, food, and medical/legal assistance

- Works with Greyhound Lines, Inc., to send kids home by bus through the Home Free program

Can I Stay In School If I Am Homeless?

Whether you are homeless along with your parents or by yourself, there are special rules schools must follow to help you stay in school or get back to school.

Chapter 57

Second Chance Homes

Second Chance Homes are adult-supervised, supportive group homes or apartment clusters for teen mothers and their children who cannot live at home because of abuse, neglect, or other extenuating circumstances. Second Chance Homes can also offer supports to help young families become self-sufficient and reduce the risk of repeat pregnancies. They provide a home where teen mothers can live, but they also offer program services to help put young mothers and their children on the path to a better future. Several federal resources are available to help state and local governments and community-based organizations create Second Chance Homes that provide safe, stable, nurturing environments for teen mothers and their children.

Second Chance Homes programs vary across the country, but generally include the following:

- An adult-supervised, supportive living arrangement
- Pregnancy prevention services or referrals
- A requirement to finish high school or obtain a GED
- Access to support services such as child care, health care, transportation, and counseling
- Parenting and life skills classes
- Education, job training, and employment services
- Community involvement

About This Chapter: Information in this chapter is from "About Second Chance Homes," and "Available Resources—Second Chance Homes," publications of the U.S. Department of Housing and Urban Development, available online through http://portal.hud.gov; accessed September 2011.

- Individual case management and mentoring

- Culturally sensitive services

- Services to ensure a smooth transition to independent living

The Importance Of Second Chance Homes

Second Chance Homes offer a nurturing home for society's most vulnerable families, teen mothers and their children with nowhere else to go. Almost half of all poor children under six are born to adolescent parents. Children of teen mothers are 50 percent more likely to have low birthweight, 33 percent more likely to become teen mothers themselves, and 2.7 times more likely to be incarcerated than the sons of mothers who delay childbearing. Teen mothers are half as likely to earn their high school diplomas or GEDs and are more likely to be on welfare than mothers who are older when they give birth. In addition, research shows that over 60 percent of teen parents have experienced sexual and/or physical abuse, often by a household member. Limited early findings indicate that residents of Second Chance Homes have fewer repeat pregnancies, better high school/GED completion rates, stronger life skills, increased self-sufficiency, and healthier babies.

Second Chance Homes help teen mothers and their children comply with welfare reform requirements. Under the 1996 welfare law, an unmarried parent under 18 cannot receive welfare assistance unless she lives with a parent, guardian, or adult relative. However, if such a living arrangement is inappropriate (for example, if her family's whereabouts are unknown or if she was abused), states may waive the rule and either determine her current living arrangement to be appropriate, or help her find an alternative adult-supervised supportive living arrangement such as a Second Chance Home. Also, in states where alternatives such as Second Chance Homes are currently not available, teen mothers could be forced to choose between inappropriate living arrangements and losing their cash assistance. Making Second Chance Homes available to teen mothers in need could provide these teens with stable housing, case management, and preparation for independent living.

Second Chance Homes can support teen families who are homeless or in foster care. State foster care systems may not have the capacity to place the teens and their children together, and frequently, homeless shelters, battered women's shelters, and transitional living facilities cannot accept teen parents under age 17. Unfortunately, homelessness poses the threat of separation in young families. For vulnerable families with no safe, stable places to go, Second Chance Homes can help fill the gap.

Eligibility

Eligibility criteria for Second Chance Homes vary from program to program. Some programs are targeted for adolescent mothers (between the ages of 14 to 20, for example), mothers receiving welfare assistance, or homeless families. Other programs are open to any mother in need of a place to live—regardless of age, income, or the assistance program for which she qualifies.

Location

Nationwide, at least six states have made a statewide commitment to Second Chance Home programs: Massachusetts, Nevada, New Mexico, Rhode Island, Texas, and Georgia. In statewide networks, community-based organizations operate the homes under contract to the states and deliver the services. States share in the cost of the program, refer teens to homes, and set standards and guidelines for services to teen families. In addition, there are many local Second Chance Home programs operating in an estimated 25 additional states.

Federal Resources

State legislatures may allocate Temporary Assistance to Needy Families (TANF) block grant funds for Second Chance Homes. Like TANF, state maintenance-of-effort (MOE) funds and the Social Services Block Grant (SSBG) are flexible, and largely under states' discretion in terms of how they are spent. States and communities may also explore other sources of funding from the U.S. Department of Health and Human Services (HHS) and the U.S. Department of Housing and Urban Development (HUD). Additional state and private sources of funding are available to fill in funding gaps, help providers acquire or rehabilitate Second Chance Homes, or develop specialized Second Chance Homes for teen parents who are homeless or in foster care.

It's A Fact!

Teen mothers can be referred to Second Chance Homes through welfare agencies, homeless shelters, or foster care programs, or by community organizations, schools, clinics, or hospitals. Mothers may also self-refer.

Source: From "About Second Chance Homes," a publication of the U.S. Department of Housing and Urban Development.

More Information

The list of available resources in this chapter contains detailed information on the major sources of federal funding for Second Chance Homes that are available from HHS and HUD. In addition to the federal sites that are included here, more general information on the program may be found at the Administration for Children and Families (the agency that oversees most of the relevant programs within the Department of Health and Human Services) and the Department of Housing and Urban Development.

HHS Sources Of Assistance

Temporary Assistance For Needy Families (TANF) Block Grant And State Maintenance Of Effort Dollars (MOE)

These funds can pay for the following:

- Planning and operating costs

- Cash assistance to teens

- Parenting and life skills classes

- Child care

- Job training and placement

- Counseling

- Case management

- Follow-up services

- Anything that reasonably meets the four broad purposes of TANF

These funds cannot be used for the following:

- Facility construction or medical care except family planning

- Assistance such as housing and cash aid can only go to needy teens.

- For MOE, all funds must be spent on needy families. States define who is needy.

States receive funds in the form of block grants; states decide how funds are spent within the context of TANF. There is a plan that must be reviewed and certified by HHS. For MOE, states decide how funds are spent.

State contacts for this funding stream are provided through the Office of Family Assistance.

> ## It's A Fact!
>
> There are a number of nongovernmental organizations that have been actively assessing Second Chance Homes and providing technical assistance to states. The Social Policy Action Network (SPAN) has been a leader in documenting existing programs, identifying best practices, and developing guides and a directory of homes. Other organizations that can provide useful information about providing services to teen parents in need include The Child Welfare League of America, Florence Crittendon Division (CWLA), the Center for Law and Social Policy (CLASP), and the Center for Assessment and Policy Development (CAPD).
>
> Source: From "About Second Chance Homes," a publication of the U.S. Department of Housing and Urban Development.

Child Care Development Fund (CCDF)

Theses funds can pay for child care assistance for low-income families who are working or attending training/education and quality improvement efforts such as grants or training for child care providers.

CCDF cannot be used for construction or major renovation (except for Indian tribes). Families receiving subsidies must meet income eligibility requirements and have children under age 13 (or age 19 if not capable of self-care).

States, territories, and Indian tribes receive CCDF in the form of formula block grants. State contacts for this funding stream are provided through the Administration for Children and Families, Child Care Bureau.

Social Services Block Grant (SSBG)

These funds can be used for the following:

- Planning and operating costs
- Parenting and life skills classes
- Child care
- Job training and placement
- Counseling
- Case management
- Follow-up services

These funds cannot be used for the following:

- Facility purchase, construction, or renovation
- Medical care except family planning
- Cash aid
- Unlicensed child care
- Drug rehab
- Public education
- Room and board
- Services in hospitals, nursing homes, or prisons

States receive funds in the form of formula block grants; states must report to HHS on how funds are spent and who is served.

Child Welfare Services Title IV-B Subpart 1 And 2 Funds

These funds can pay for child welfare services, family preservation and reunification, family support, and adoption promotion and support. All children receiving state or federal foster care funds must also receive certain protections under Title IV-B. States and Indian tribes receive Title IV-B subpart 1 and 2 funds on a formula basis. You can get more information on this type of funding from the Children's Bureau Programs.

Independent Living Program

These funds can pay for room and board (for youth aged 18–21 only); education; life skills training; counseling; and case management. Funds must be spent on youth between the ages of 18 and 21 to assist them in making the transition from foster care to independent living.

States receive these funds on a formula basis. You can get more information on these funds from the Children's Bureau Programs.

Transitional Living Program For Homeless Youth

These funds can be used for housing, life skills training, interpersonal skills building, education, job training, and health care. Funds can only be used to serve youth aged 16–21 for up to 18 months who are homeless, including those for whom it is not possible to live in a safe environment with a relative and who do not have an alternative safe living arrangement.

HHS awards three-year competitive grants to multi-purpose youth service organizations. You can get more information about these funds from the Transitional Living Program for Homeless Youth (TLP).

HUD Sources Of Assistance

Community Development Block Grant (CDBG)

These funds can be used for the following:

- Facility purchase, construction, or renovation
- Planning operating costs
- Parenting and life skills classes
- Child care
- Job training and placement
- Counseling
- Case management
- Follow-up services

At least 70 percent of funds must benefit low and moderate income families; states and communities must prepare an action plan with community input. States, major cities, and urban counties receive these funds in the form of formula block grants. Contact your local HUD office for more information.

HUD Supportive Housing Program

These funds can be used for the following:

- Facility purchase, construction, or renovation
- New or increased services to the homeless
- Operating expenses
- Some administrative costs

Funds must be spent on homeless persons only; 25 percent must be set aside for families with children; 25 percent must be set aside for disabled; 10 percent must be set aside for supportive services not provided with housing. Homeless minors may be eligible to receive services under this funding source unless they are considered wards of the state under applicable state law.

HUD awards three-year, renewable competitive grants to states, tribes, cities, counties, other governmental entities, private nonprofits, and community mental health associations. Contact your local HUD office for more information.

HUD Emergency Shelter Grants

These funds can be used for the following:

- Facility renovation

- Operating costs

- Homelessness prevention

- Employment, health, drug abuse, and education services

Funds must be spent on the homeless or those at risk of being homeless; only five percent of funds can be used for administrative costs, and 30 percent for prevention and services. Homeless minors may be eligible to receive services under this funding source unless they are considered wards of the state under applicable state law.

States, major cities, and urban counties receive these funds in the form of formula grants. Contact your local HUD office for more information.

Rental Assistance Vouchers

In general, the voucher pays the landlord the difference between 30 percent of a renting family's gross income and the price of the rental unit, up to a local maximum.

In order to receive a voucher, a renter must apply to his/her local Public Housing Authority. Contact your local Public Housing Authority for more information.

It's A Fact!

Teenage mothers may be eligible for rental assistance vouchers. However, the voucher program requires that a lease be signed by the renter, and in some states minors may not sign a lease. Individual Public Housing Authorities (PHAs) determine whether a shared housing facility is an acceptable use for the voucher. The PHA must approve the renter and the unit according to various eligibility criteria.

Source: From "Available Resources—Second Chance Homes," a publication of the U.S. Department of Housing and Urban Development.

HUD's Dollar Homes Program

These funds can be used for property acquisition. Local governments (cities and counties) can purchase HUD owned homes for $1 each, plus closing costs, to create housing for families and communities in need. Local governments can purchase these homes and then convey them to nonprofit organizations for use.

HUD's NonProfit Sales Program

These funds can be used for property acquisition. Nonprofit organizations can purchase properties at a discount through this program. The funds cannot be used for direct sales of properties foreclosed by the Federal Housing Authority. Discounts of 30 percent off the list price are offered if the property is not eligible for FHA insurance and is located in a HUD-designated revitalization area. Other properties are offered at 10 percent discounts off list price (or 15 percent if five or more properties are purchased and closed in a single transaction). These discounts apply to sales in both restricted and general property listings.

Other Sources Of Assistance

McKinney Act Title V Program

These funds can be used for property acquisition. Properties are leased without charge for a period of one to 20 years, but the entity providing homeless services must pay for operating and repair costs. Surplus properties can be made available to states, local governments, and nonprofit organizations to assist the homeless. Available properties are listed in the HUD Federal Register notice listing property availability. HHS handles the application portion of the program.

Military Base Closures

These funds can be used for property acquisition. When a military base is being closed, a Local Redevelopment Authority is designated to redeploy the assets of the base.

Chapter 58

Health Insurance Options For Women

What is health insurance?

Health insurance is a formal agreement to provide and/or pay for medical care. The health insurance policy describes what medical services are covered by the insurance company. There are medical services that are not covered and will not be paid by your insurance company.

There are a variety of private and public health insurance programs. Most women obtain health insurance through their employer or as a dependent in a family plan. There also are public health insurance plans funded by the federal and state governments.

How does health insurance affect me?

More than 17 million women (nearly one in five) aged 18 to 64 are uninsured in the United States. As health insurance costs soar, employers cut benefits, or jobs disappear, millions of people slip through the cracks and lose their coverage. These are working Americans who make too much money to qualify for Medicaid, but don't have enough money to buy health insurance. Also, women are twice as likely as men to be insured as a dependent on a spouse's plan. So, she risks losing coverage if she divorces, is widowed, or if her spouse loses his job.

What are my health care options?

Health insurance can be complicated and confusing. There are different types of plans.

Private Health Insurance: There are two major types of private health insurance:

About This Chapter: Information in this chapter is from "Health insurance and women fact sheet," a publication of the Office on Women's Health, U.S. Department of Health and Human Services, July 2007.

- **Fee-For-Service:** The provider (such as a doctor or hospital) gets paid for each covered service. With this type, you go to a doctor of your choice, then the doctor or hospital submits a claim to your insurance company for payment. The insurance company will only pay the provider for covered services. Most fee-for-service plans have a deductible amount that you must pay each year before the insurance company will begin to pay for medical services. Many plans also require you to pay a portion of the medical expense—called coinsurance.

- **Managed Care:** Managed care plans have contracts with certain doctors, hospitals, and other providers to provide medical services to plan members. The three main types of managed care plans are the following:

  - **Health Maintenance Organizations (HMOs):** They provide health services for a fixed monthly payment, called a premium. This monthly premium is the same whether you use the plan's services or not. The plan may charge a copayment for some services—for example $10 for an office visit or $5 for a prescription. HMO plans usually require you to select a primary care physician (PCP), who manages your care. As long as you use the doctors and hospitals that participate in the HMO, your out-of-pocket costs should be very small. The HMO Act of 1973 created this alternative to traditional health plans as a more affordable option.

  - **Preferred Provider Organization (PPO):** This option offers more choices than an HMO, but premiums often are higher. Most PPO plans do not require you to have a PCP to manage your care. You can keep your out-of-pocket costs low by using in-network providers.

  - **Point Of Service (POS):** This plan is similar to a PPO, but your care is managed by a PCP. For example, with a POS plan, you would need a referral from your PCP to see a specialist.

People who have private insurance either buy it themselves or get it through their employer, called group insurance. Group insurance obtained through an employer typically requires the employee to pay some of the overall policy cost.

Public Health Insurance: The government also provides health care coverage for qualifying women through Medicaid, Medicare, and special interest programs. These plans serve those who meet certain financial, age, or situational requirements. Government health insurance programs include the following:

- **Medicare:** This is the national health insurance program for people age 65 or older, under age 65 with certain disabilities, and any age with permanent kidney failure. How you get your health care coverage depends on the Medicare plan you select.

- **Medicaid:** Medicaid provides health care to certain low-income individuals and families with limited resources. Medicaid does not pay money to you. Instead, it sends payments directly to your health care providers. Medicaid is a state and federally funded program. Although the federal government sets general program rules, each state defines its own eligibility rules and runs its own program services. Qualification in one state does not mean you will qualify in another state. You must be a U.S. national, citizen, or permanent resident alien in order to apply for benefits.

- **State Children's Health Insurance Program (SCHIP):** This is a joint state and federal program that provides insurance for children of qualifying families. Families who make too much money to qualify for Medicaid but cannot afford private health insurance may be able to qualify for SCHIP assistance. Eligibility and health care coverage varies according to each state.

How do I choose a health plan?

When it comes to health plans, not everyone has a choice. But if you do, you will need to understand how different plans affect your choice of providers and services, costs, and quality of care. This information can be confusing.

It's A Fact!

Many states have become more flexible in their ability to serve families in need, especially if you fall into any of the following categories:

- **Pregnant:** Both you and your child will be covered if you qualify.
- **Children/Teenagers:** May cover sick children or teenagers on their own.
- **Aged, Blind, And/Or Disabled:** Nursing home and hospice care available.
- **Leaving Welfare:** You may be able to get temporary assistance.

Call your local social security office for more information.

I don't have health insurance. What are my options?

There are a number of resources for women without health insurance. There are government-sponsored safety-net facilities that provide medical care for those in need, even if they have no insurance or money. Safety-net facilities include community health centers, public hospitals, school-based centers, public housing primary care centers, migrant health centers, and special needs facilities. To find a facility near you, contact your local or state health department or visit the Bureau of Primary Health Care.

Other government-sponsored programs for uninsured women include:

- **Special Supplemental Nutrition Program For Women, Infants, And Children (WIC):** Provides healthy foods to supplement diets, nutrition education, and referrals to health care for low-income women, infants, and children up to age five.

- **Maternal And Child Health Services (MCH):** State programs provide health care services for low-income women who are pregnant and their children under age 22. The federal government funds these programs and establishes general guidelines regarding services. Each state determines eligibility and identifies the specific services to be provided. The Title V State MCH Toll-free Hotline Directory can help you find services in your state.

What if I do not qualify for these government programs?

Some uninsured women make too much money to qualify for government assistance but cannot afford to pay for health insurance or costly medical care. This is a difficult situation for women and their families. There are options for women in this situation, including the following:

- **Free Clinics:** Free clinics provide services for the working poor and uninsured. Usually, people who qualify for Medicare or Medicaid or who can afford private insurance do not qualify for care in free clinics. The Free Clinic Foundation of America publishes a National Directory of Free Clinics. To access the directory, visit www.medkind.com.

- **Prescription Drug Assistance:** Some states provide prescription drug assistance to women who are not covered by Medicaid. Also, many drug companies will work with your doctor or health care provider to supply free medicines to those in need.

- **Women With Cancer:** Women who are coping with cancer can find help through many government-sponsored and volunteer organizations.

- **Women With Human Immunodeficiency Virus (HIV):** The federal Ryan White CARE Act funds services for those with HIV/acquired immune deficiency syndrome

(AIDS) who have little or no insurance and limited income. For information about the Ryan White CARE Act, go to http://hab.hrsa.gov. Contact your local or state health department to locate a CARE provider in your area. Resources also can be found at www.aids.gov.

- **Low-Cost Health Insurance Options:** Some labor unions, professional clubs, associations, and organizations offer private group health insurance to members. These plans usually are less costly and may be an option to consider.

- **State Temporary Insurance:** Some who have been denied health insurance because of a medical condition may be able to obtain coverage through State High Risk Pools. More than 30 states provide this temporary insurance assistance.

Chapter 59

WIC: The Special Supplemental Nutrition Program For Women, Infants, And Children

What is WIC?

WIC provides nutritious foods, nutrition education, and referrals to health and other social services to participants at no charge. WIC serves low-income pregnant, postpartum, and breastfeeding women, and infants and children up to age five who are at nutrition risk.

Where is WIC available?

The program is available in all 50 States, 34 Indian Tribal Organizations, American Samoa, District of Columbia, Guam, Commonwealth Islands of the Northern Marianas, Puerto Rico, and the Virgin Islands. These 90 WIC state agencies administer the program through approximately 2,200 local agencies and 9,000 clinic sites.

Who is eligible?

Women who are pregnant or postpartum, infants, and children up to age five are eligible. They must meet income guidelines and a state residency requirement, and be individually determined to be at nutrition risk by a health professional.

To be eligible on the basis of income, applicants' income must fall at or below 185 percent of the U.S. Poverty Income Guidelines (currently $40,793 for a family of four). A person who participates or has family members who participate in certain other benefit programs, such as the Supplemental Nutrition Assistance Program, Medicaid, or Temporary Assistance for Needy Families, automatically meets the income eligibility requirement.

About This Chapter: Information in this chapter is from "WIC: The Special Supplemental Nutrition Program for Women, Infants, and Children," a publication of the U.S. Department of Agriculture, November 2009.

It's A Fact!

WIC is not an entitlement program; i.e., Congress does not set aside funds to allow every eligible individual to participate in the program. Instead, WIC is a federal grant program for which Congress authorizes a specific amount of funding each year for program operations. The Food and Nutrition Service, which administers the program at the federal level, provides these funds to WIC state agencies (State health departments or comparable agencies) to pay for WIC foods, nutrition education, breastfeeding promotion and support, and administrative costs.

What is nutrition risk?

Two major types of nutrition risk are recognized for WIC eligibility:

- Medically-based risks such as anemia, underweight, overweight, history of pregnancy complications, or poor pregnancy outcomes.

- Dietary risks, such as failure to meet the dietary guidelines or inappropriate nutrition practices.

Nutrition risk is determined by a health professional such as a physician, nutritionist, or nurse, and is based on federal guidelines. This health screening is free to program applicants.

How many people does WIC serve?

During the final quarter of Fiscal Year (FY) 2009, the number of women, infants, and children receiving WIC benefits each month reached approximately 9.3 million. In 1974, the first year WIC was permanently authorized, 88,000 people participated. By 1980, participation was at 1.9 million; by 1985, 3.1 million; by 1990, 4.5 million; and by 2000, 7.2 million. Average monthly participation for FY 2008 was approximately 8.7 million.

Children have always been the largest category of WIC participants. Of the 8.7 million people who received WIC benefits each month in FY 2008, approximately 4.33 million were children, 2.22 million were infants, and 2.15 million were women.

What food benefits do WIC participants receive?

In most WIC state agencies, WIC participants receive checks or vouchers to purchase specific foods each month that are designed to supplement their diets with specific nutrients that benefit WIC's target population. In addition, some states issue an electronic benefit card to participants instead of paper checks or vouchers. The use of electronic cards is expected to grow as Food and

Nutrition Service (FNS) is promoting WIC electronic benefit transfer (EBT) nationwide. A few state agencies distribute the WIC foods through warehouses or deliver the foods to participants' homes. Different food packages are provided for different categories of participants.

WIC foods include infant cereal, iron-fortified adult cereal, vitamin C-rich fruit or vegetable juice, eggs, milk, cheese, peanut butter, dried and canned beans/peas, and canned fish. Soy-based beverages, tofu, fruits and vegetables, baby foods, whole wheat bread, and other whole-grain options were recently added to better meet the nutritional needs of WIC participants.

WIC recognizes and promotes breastfeeding as the optimal source of nutrition for infants. For women who do not fully breastfeed, WIC provides iron-fortified infant formula. Special infant formulas and medical foods may be provided when prescribed by a physician for a specified medical condition.

Who gets first priority for participation?

If WIC cannot serve all the eligible people who apply for benefits, a system of priorities has been established for filling program openings. Once a local WIC agency has reached its maximum caseload, vacancies are filled in the order of the following priority levels:

- Pregnant women, breastfeeding women, and infants determined to be at nutrition risk because of a nutrition-related medical condition.

- Infants up to six months of age whose mothers participated in WIC or could have participated and had a medical problem.

- Children at nutrition risk because of a nutrition-related medical problem.

- Pregnant or breastfeeding women and infants at nutrition risk because of an inadequate dietary pattern.

- Children at nutrition risk because of an inadequate dietary pattern.

- Nonbreastfeeding, postpartum women with any nutrition risk.

- Individuals at nutrition risk only because they are homeless or migrants, and current participants who, without WIC foods, could continue to have medical and/or dietary problems.

How does WIC support breastfeeding?

Since a major goal of the WIC Program is to improve the nutritional status of infants, WIC mothers are encouraged to breastfeed their infants, unless medically contraindicated.

- WIC mothers who breastfeed their infants are provided information and support through counseling and breastfeeding educational materials.

- Breastfeeding mothers receive a greater quantity and variety of foods than mothers who fully formula feed their infants, with mothers fully breastfeeding their infants receiving the most substantial food package.

- Breastfeeding mothers are eligible to participate in WIC longer than nonbreastfeeding mothers.

- Breastfeeding mothers may receive follow-up support through peer counselors.

- Breastfeeding mothers may receive breast pumps and other aides to help support the initiation and continuation of breastfeeding.

What is the WIC infant formula rebate system?

Mothers participating in WIC are encouraged to breastfeed their infants if possible, but WIC state agencies provide infant formula for mothers who choose to use this feeding method. WIC state agencies are required by law to have competitively bid infant formula rebate contracts with infant formula manufacturers. This means WIC state agencies agree to provide one brand of infant formula and in return the manufacturer gives the state agency a rebate for each can of infant formula purchased by WIC participants. The brand of infant formula provided by WIC varies from state agency to state agency depending on which company has the rebate contract in a particular state.

By negotiating rebates with formula manufacturers, states are able to serve more people. For fiscal year 2008, rebate savings were $2.0 billion, supporting an average of 2.14 million participants each month, or 25 percent of the estimated average monthly caseload.

What is WIC's current funding level?

Congress appropriated $7.252 billion for WIC in fiscal year 2010. By comparison, the WIC Program appropriation was $20.6 million in 1974; $750 million in 1980; $1.5 billion in 1985; $2.1 billion in 1990, and $4.0 billion in 2000.

It's A Fact!

Information on food and nutrition service (FNS) programs is available on the world wide web at www.fns.usda.gov/fns.

Chapter 60

Vaccines For Uninsured Children

The Vaccines for Children (VFC) Program helps provide vaccines to children whose parents or guardians may not be able to afford them. This helps ensure that all children have a better chance of getting their recommended vaccinations on schedule. These vaccines protect babies, young children, and adolescents from 16 diseases.

Who is eligible for the VFC Program?

Your child is eligible for the VFC Program if he or she is younger than 19 years of age and is one of the following:

- Medicaid eligible
- Uninsured
- Underinsured
- American Indian or Alaska Native

What is underinsured?

Underinsured means your child has health insurance, but the insurance deals with vaccines in one of the following ways:

- Doesn't cover vaccines
- Doesn't cover certain vaccines

About This Chapter: Information in this chapter is from "VFC Program: Vaccines for Uninsured Children," a publication of the Centers for Disease Control and Prevention, January 2011.

> ## It's A Fact!
>
> Vaccines available through the VFC Program are those recommended by the Advisory Committee on Immunization Practices (ACIP) and approved by the Centers for Disease Control and Prevention (CDC). CDC, as the administrator of VFC, purchases and distributes the vaccines to private and public health care providers who are enrolled in the VFC Program.

- Covers vaccines but has a fixed dollar limit or cap for vaccines. Once that fixed dollar amount is reached, your child is then eligible.

Underinsured children are eligible to receive vaccines only at Federally Qualified Health Centers (FQHC) or Rural Health Clinics (RHC). An FQHC is a type of provider that meets certain criteria under Medicare and Medicaid programs. If you need help locating an FQHC or RHC, contact your state VFC coordinator.

What is the cost?

There is no charge for any vaccines given by a VFC provider to eligible children. But there can be some other costs with a vaccination:

- Doctors can charge a set (or standard) fee to administer each shot. But if the family can't afford the fee per shot, the fee must be excused. A VFC-eligible child cannot be refused a vaccination due to the parent's or guardian's inability to pay for shot administration.

- There can be a fee for the office visit.

- There can be fees for non-vaccine services, like an eye exam or blood test.

> ## It's A Fact!
>
> If your child's doctor isn't a VFC provider, you can take your child to one of the following places to get VFC vaccinations:
>
> - Public health clinic (local health department)
> - Federally Qualified Health Center (FQHC)
> - Rural Health Clinic (RHC)
>
> The best place to take your child depends on where you live and what type of eligibility your child has under the VFC Program. Contact your state's VFC Coordinator to find out where to take your child for VFC vaccinations.

Where can my child get vaccinated?

If your child is eligible, check that your child's doctor is a VFC Program provider.

You can find your state's VFC Coordinator online. Or call 1-800-CDC-INFO (232-4636) and ask for the phone number of your state's VFC Coordinator.

Who funds and manages the VFC Progam?

The VFC Program is funded by the United States government. In general, state health departments manage the VFC Program, but in some locations it may be managed by a city or territorial health department. Nationwide, there are over 40,000 doctors enrolled in the VFC Program.

What diseases do the recommended vaccines protect against?

- Diphtheria
- Haemophilus influenzae type b (Hib)
- Hepatitis A
- Hepatitis B
- Human Papillomavirus (HPV)
- Influenza (flu)
- Measles
- Meningococcal disease
- Mumps
- Pertussis (whooping cough)
- Pneumococcal disease
- Polio
- Rotavirus
- Rubella (German measles)
- Tetanus (lockjaw)
- Varicella (chickenpox)

Chapter 61

Understanding Child Care Options

What types of child care are there?

Not all child care programs are the same. Different families have different needs. Below you will find various descriptions of child care programs. Your local Child Care Resource and Referral (CCR & R) will work with you to determine what programs are available in your area.

- **Child Care Center:** A nonresidential program, often with children separated by classrooms or age groups. Child care centers have program directors, lead teachers and assistant teachers, and additional staff. Child care centers are likely to offer children a structured curriculum.

- **Family Child Care Home:** Child care offered in a provider's home. You see more mixed ages in a Family Child Care setting. Staff includes the provider/owner and maybe one or two additional staff. Family Child Care providers may or may not offer a structured curriculum.

- **Preschool/PreK/Prekindergarten:** An early education program for children ages three to five. Preschool programs offer curriculum to help your child prepare for school. Some child care programs may refer to the three to five year old classroom as the PreK classroom.

  - **Part-Day Preschool:** A program two to three hours a day, for three to five days a week. These programs focus on early education and school readiness. With a part-day preschool program, you may need to look for additional child care options to accommodate your work schedule and the schedule of the program. These programs may be available to all families.

About This Chapter: Information in this chapter is excerpted from "Putting the pieces together... solving the childcare puzzle," © 2010 National Association of Child Care Resource & Referral Agencies (NACCRRA), www .naccrra.org. All rights reserved. Reprinted with permission.

- **State-Funded Prekindergarten Programs:** Programs targeting children ages three to five, focusing on early education and school readiness. Some states offer these programs at either a low or no cost to eligible families. Programs may be part day or a full school day. With a state-funded prekindergarten program, you may need to look for additional child care options to accommodate your work schedule and the schedule of the program.

*It is always important to clarify what a particular programs means when someone refers to "PreK".

- **Head Start Programs:** Child development programs funded by the U.S. Department of Health and Human Services. These comprehensive programs offer an educational setting, health and nutrition information, and various parent involvement opportunities. Head Start programs typically have income eligibility guidelines.

- **Inclusive Child Care:** Programs that offer child care services to families of children with special needs. These programs strive to keep all children in a common environment or classroom. Inclusive programs eliminate the separation of typically developing children and children with special needs.

What age group is your child in?

In different child care settings, the age of your child may determine what classroom or group he is in. It may also affect the amount you pay for child care. It is good to familiarize yourself with these age classifications.

- **Infants:** Birth to age 12–18 months (may vary by setting)
- **Toddlers:** 12–18 months to 36 months
- **Preschoolers:** 3–5 years old
- **School-age:** 5–12 years old

What help is available to pay for child care?

At times, you may find yourself looking for help with your child care payments. Financial assistance options vary by location, but here are some examples that may be available to you.

- **State Programs:** Federally funded financial assistance programs, or subsidy programs, that pay a portion of an eligible family's child care fees. These programs are offered by state agencies and distributed through state or local programs. Income eligibility requirements vary by state.

- **Local Programs:** In some areas, there may be local programs available to your family that will assist with your child care costs. Programs may be offered through local governments, nonprofit agencies, or service organizations.

- **Employer Programs:** Some employers may offer child care assistance through Dependant Care assistance accounts or other Employee Assistance Programs.

- **Provider Specific Programs:** Child care programs may offer financial assistance for families. Incentives to ask a prospective provider about include sliding fee scales, scholarships, or sibling discounts.

- **Tax Credits:** There are various tax credits your family might be eligible for if you have qualifying children. Visit www.irs.gov for specific information.

  - Earned Income Tax Credit
  - Child Tax Credit
  - Child and Dependent Care Tax Credit
  - State Tax Credits

Why is screening important?

When you return to work or school, you want to know that you have selected the most suitable child care environment for your child. By screening prospective child care programs, you will have done your homework and made an informed child care choice.

- **Interview:** Visit with prospective child care providers and/or center directors and teachers. Get to know a little bit more about who will be caring for your child.

- **On-Site Visit:** Be sure to visit the child care program. You may visit more than once. You might want to visit one on one with the provider. You will also want to visit with children present. You will be able to observe caregiver and child interactions.

- **Training:** Learn about the training prospective providers have gone through to become a caregiver. Also ask about ongoing training opportunities.

- **Background Checks:** Check with both child care centers and family child care providers regarding the completion of background check on all individuals/staff that will have contact with your child.

- **References:** Speak to other families, both past and current, about their experiences in the program.

Who regulates child care?

Regulations for child care vary from state to state. Each state has a regulatory agency that oversees the implementation and compliance of standards and guidelines set for local child care providers. In addition, child care providers and centers can voluntarily go through programs focusing on the quality of care being offered to families.

- **Licensed:** States have regulations in place for licensing child care centers and family child care homes. It is important that you check to see what the regulations are in your state. Your local Child Care Resource and Referral agency will be able to assist you with this information.

- **Licensed-Exempt:** In some states, certain types of programs are not required to be licensed. These programs may include family child care homes with six or fewer children, religious-based child care programs, and programs offered in public schools.

- **Accreditation:** A voluntary program requiring child care providers to meet specific nationally recognized performance standards. These standards generally exceed state licensing requirements. Some accrediting organizations include:

  - National Association for the Education of Young Children (NAEYC) www.naeyc.org

  - National Accreditation Commission for Early Care and Education Programs (NAC) www.naccp.org

  - National Early Childhood Program Accreditation (NECPA) www.necpa.net

  - National Association of Family Child Care (NAFCC) www.nafcc.org

  - Council on Accreditation (COA) www.coanet.org

- **Quality Rating And Improvement Systems (QRIS):** Statewide or local programs created to improve the quality and affordability of child care. The focus of these programs is consumer education benchmarks and tiered reimbursement programs.

Now that you are prepared to begin your search for child care, keep in mind the choices you make will impact your child's future. Your child care provider will work with you as your child's nurturer, educator, and cheerleader when you are not there to care for your child. Maintaining a solid, consistent, long-term relationship will positively impact your child's early experiences and preparation for school.

What are you looking for?

There are many terms associated with the full- or part-time care of your child. Most commonly, you might hear "child care" or "day care."

- **Child Care, Day Care, Early Care, And Education Programs:** Full-time care and supervision of your child(ren), typically between 6:00 a.m. and 6:00 p.m. These programs offer safe, structured learning environments that help prepare your child for school.

- **Babysitter:** Care offered on an as-needed basis through a friend, neighbor, or young adult in your area. You may look for a babysitter when you need to run an errand in the evening or on the weekend.

It's A Fact!

Use the tips below to familiarize a babysitter with safety and first aid:

- Ask if the babysitter knows infant/child cardiopulmonary resuscitation (CPR) and first aid.
- Remind the babysitter that infants should not be placed on an adult bed of any kind.
- Remind the babysitter to place the baby on her/his back to sleep.
- Be sure that the babysitter knows the signs of illness in an infant including: changes in skin color, sweating, nausea or vomiting, and diarrhea.
- Show the babysitter where the fire extinguishers are kept, and explain how they are used.
- Be sure to show the babysitter where the first aid supplies are kept.
- Remind the babysitter to keep all balloons or plastic items away from the baby.
- Tell the babysitter that children should never be left alone in the bathtub. The sitter should always bring along the children should she or he need to leave the room, such as to answer the telephone or the door bell.
- Remind the babysitter to keep the bathroom door closed and the toilet seat and lid down when not in use.

Use the tips below to familiarize the babysitter with your house:

- Be sure to give the babysitter a tour of the house.
- Ensure that all windows have been closed and that the babysitter knows to keep them closed.
- Show the babysitter how to operate your child safety gates and where they go.
- Show the babysitter where the flashlights are located.
- Make sure that you have put away all sharp items including scissors, knives, and any other objects that can cause injury.

Source: From "Babysitters and child care," a publication of the Office on Women's Health, U.S. Department of Health and Human Services, September 2010.

When do you need child care?

Families' schedules vary. You know best when you will need child care to accommodate everyone's schedule.

- **Traditional Hours:** Traditional hours include the 8:00 a.m. to 5:00 p.m. work day, with time allotted for pick up and drop off. Generally a child care program offering care during traditional hours might be open from 6:00 a.m. to 6:00 p.m.

- **Nontraditional Hours:** This type of care may be more appealing to shift workers and families needing child care in the evenings and on the weekends. Nontraditional hours may include overnight or after-hours care.

- **Irregular Duty:** Families needing care for irregular duty may need a child care provider who can accommodate their nontraditional work schedule. Examples of irregular duty may include a rotating schedule with four days on shift, four days off shift.

Chapter 62

Finding Help Paying For Child Care

Five Steps To Healthy Child Care Budgeting

1. Plan Ahead

Start thinking about child care options and cost as far in advance as you can. No matter what type of care you are considering—a child care center, care in someone's home, or care for an infant, toddler, preschooler, or school-age child—finding the right child care option or help with child care expenses can take some time.

2. Call The Experts

Begin the search by calling your local experts—your Child Care Resource and Referral agency (CCR&R). CCR&Rs can give you the facts about child care. They can also provide a list of child care options and available financial assistance in your area.

3. Be A Smart Consumer

When you are at work, you want to know that your child is getting the kind of high-quality care that all children need to be healthy, happy, and ready for school.

The Check It Out checklist in this chapter helps you evaluate the value of the child care you are buying for your family. You can use this checklist in a child care center, a family child care home (care in someone else's home), or for an in-home provider who comes to your home.

About This Chapter: Information in this chapter is excerpted from "Finding Help Paying for Child Care," © 2009 National Association of Child Care Resource & Referral Agencies (NACCRRA), www.naccrra.org. All rights reserved. Reprinted with permission.

> ## Quick Tip
> Call 1-800-424-2246 or visit ChildCareAware.org to find the CCR&R in your area.

The money you pay goes toward the caregivers' salary and ongoing education and training so they can meet your child's needs. Your child care fees also help purchase food, toys, equipment, and supplies, and pay for insurance, rent or mortgage, and other necessary expenses.

Once you have evaluated your options and decided on a child care setting, be an involved and informed consumer. Visit often and participate in events at your child's program. This sends a strong message to your child and your child's provider that you think what your child is doing and learning is important.

4. Find Out What Kind Of Help May Be Available

The following child care assistance programs help families with the high cost of child care. Each type of child care financial assistance has different qualifications, so work with your local CCR&R and your employer's human resources department to make sure you get all the facts.

- **State Child Care Subsidies:** Child care subsidies are available in every state to help families with the cost of child care. Usually, child care subsidies are available for working families earning low incomes, receiving Temporary Assistance for Needy Families (TANF), or in some cases enrolled in school. If eligible, you will pay part of the cost while the rest is paid directly to your selected child care provider.

- **Local Programs:** Local government, United Way agencies, or other community or faith-based organizations sometimes provide child care scholarships.

- **Employer/College Support:** Your employer may provide child care scholarships, discounts to certain programs, or onsite child care at reduced rates. Colleges or universities may also have programs to help with child care costs.

- **Child Care Program Assistance:** Your child care provider may offer scholarships, discounts, or a sliding fee scale.

- **Pre-Kindergarten (Pre-K) Programs:** Many states offer free or low-cost prekindergarten programs for three- and four- year-old children. Eligibility requirements vary by state but the goal of all prekindergarten programs is to make sure that children are prepared for kindergarten. Public schools and other child care settings offer prekindergarten programs during school hours.

- **Head Start And Early Head Start:** Head Start and Early Head Start are federally- and sometimes state-funded full- or part-day programs that provide free early education and other services to help meet the health and school readiness needs of children in income eligible families.

- **Federal Earned Income Tax Credit (EITC):** You may be able to lower your taxes and even get money back if you qualify for the EITC. To qualify, you must be working full- or part-time and make less than a certain amount based on family size. You do not have to owe any taxes to get a refund using EITC.

- **Federal Child Tax Credit (CTC):** If you have a dependent child under age 17, you may be eligible for the Child Tax Credit, which can be worth hundreds of dollars per child. The income eligibility for the CTC is much higher than for the Earned Income Tax Credit, but you still do not have to owe any taxes to use the Child Tax Credit.

- **Federal Child And Dependent Care Tax Credit:** If you have a child under the age of 13, pay for child care, and owe federal income taxes, you may be eligible for this tax credit.

- **State Earned Income And Dependent Care Tax Credits:** Many states offer their own earned Income or Child and Dependent Care tax credits. These credits are similar to the federal ones. In some states, you do not have to owe any taxes to get the State Child and Dependent Care credit. You can get both federal and state Earned Income and Child and Dependent Care credits.

- **Dependent Care Assistance Programs (DCAPs):** Your employer may offer a Dependent Care Assistance Program, which allows you to have up to $5,000 a year deducted from your paycheck on a pre-tax basis. The money is placed in a special account to be used for child care tuition reimbursement. You should never put more money in this account than you will actually spend because you will lose unspent funds at the end of the year. You cannot claim any money you put in a DCAP for the Child and Dependent Care Tax Credit.

5. Consider All Options

Think about what your family needs and take a close look at your budget. Are there alternatives to paying full-time child care? Is it possible or desirable to work fewer hours? If you are in a two-parent household, can you work at different times and share some hours of child care? Could you share child care expenses with another family?

The most important thing is that your family and child are healthy and happy. By planning, getting the facts, and using all available resources—especially your local CCR&R—you are off to a good start in making the best choice for your family.

Check It Out

Ask these questions to evaluate your child care options:

- Does the person who will be caring for your child have special training in early childhood education, First Aid, and cardiopulmonary resuscitation (CPR)?
- How long has the child care provider been providing child care?
- If there is more than one child care provider in the setting, is the total number of children in the group still small (group size)?
- Is one child care provider caring for just a few children (low child/adult ratio)?
- If you are considering a more formal child care program, is it state licensed or regulated? Is it nationally accredited?
- Have satisfactory criminal history background checks been conducted on each adult present?
- Has the program been inspected by the licensing agency within the last 12 months?
- Does the child care provider welcome drop-in visits, parent ideas, and involvement?
- Does the child care provider get on the children's eye level to talk with them and give them lots of attention and encouragement?
- Are there planned activities for children to do as well as lots of time for free play?
- Are materials—such as books, blocks, toys and art supplies—available to children all day long?
- Does the place look clean and safe and does everyone wash his or her hands often?
- Does the child care provider have written policies and procedures, including emergency plans?
- Does the child care provider have references?
- You know your child best—will your child be happy there?

Quick Tip

Visit ChildCareAware.org or call 1-800-424-2246 for more information on financial assistance and other child care and parenting resources.

Chapter 63

Child Custody

What types of custody are there?

There are two types of custody:

- Physical custody
- Legal custody

Physical custody refers to the physical possession and control of the child.

Legal custody refers to the right to make major decisions (such as educational, medical, religious) on behalf of the child.

There are four types of physical custody:

- Primary
- Partial
- Visitation
- Shared

Primary physical custody refers to the party with whom the child primarily resides.

Partial physical custody refers to the right of the other party to take the child away from the primary custodian (usually for nights, weekends, vacations, etc.).

About This Chapter: Information in this chapter is from "Child Custody," a Consumer Legal Information Pamphlet from the Pennsylvania Bar Association, © Pennsylvania Bar Association, Revised 07/05. All Rights Reserved. Reprinted with permission. This pamphlet has been issued to inform and not to advise. It is based on Pennsylvania law. The statements are general, and individual facts in a given case may alter their application or involve other laws not referred to here. For additional pamphlets and information, visit www.pabar.org or call 800-932-0311. Editor's Note: Despite the older date of this document, readers will still find useful information about the issues related to child custody.

Visitation is the right of a parent to visit (usually supervised) with the child at the child's primary residence or another location, but does not include the right to remove the child from the primary custodian's control.

Shared custody is when the parents alternate physical custody of the children to assure regular, frequent contact with both parents.

Legal custody is most often shared between the parents, as both parents should consult before making major decisions on behalf of the child. It is rare that one parent is granted sole legal custody of a child.

It's A Fact!

Special Note: This information has been issued to inform and not to advise. It is based on Pennsylvania law. The statements are general, and individual facts in a given case may alter their application or involve other laws not referred to here.

Do I have to consult the noncustodial parent before I make decisions?

When making major decisions on behalf of the child, the noncustodial parent must be consulted if there is an order giving the parents shared legal custody of the child. Even if there is no custody order, the noncustodial parent should be consulted; major decisions should be made by the parents together. If the parents are unable to make a decision concerning a major issue, either parent may file a petition seeking an order from the court.

Each parent is permitted to make normal day-to-day decisions on behalf of the child, while the child is in the parent's physical custody.

Does the noncustodial parent have access to the child's medical and school records?

Each parent is entitled to be provided access to the child's medical, dental, school, and religious records. There is an exception in certain abuse cases when the child's address needs to remain private.

Is there a relationship between seeing the children and paying child support?

Even if a parent is not complying with a support order, if there is a custody order allowing him/her to see the child, the parent must be permitted to exercise custody of the child. If there is a problem with the support, the parent should file a support complaint, a petition to modify, or a contempt petition.

If a person who is obligated to pay support is not seeing the child, the person must still pay support. If there is a problem with the custody, the parent should file a custody complaint, a petition to modify or a petition for contempt.

When is a custody order modifiable?

A custody order is modifiable when a change in the custody arrangement is in the best interest of the child. There need not be a specific change of circumstances. The parent seeking to modify the order must show why the present order is no longer in the child's best interest.

What if the custodial parent wants to move from the area with the child?

If there is a custody order in effect, the parent seeking to move with the child must file a petition for permission to relocate the child and, if the terms of the custody order must change, a petition to modify custody.

If there is no custody order in effect, the parent with whom the child lives should notify the other parent within a reasonable amount of time of the desire to move. If the noncustodial parent objects, the custodial parent will have to file a complaint for custody and a petition to relocate.

Before the child is permitted to move, a hearing must be held as to whether the move is in the child's best interest. The burden of proof is on the parent seeking to move the child. When deciding whether the move is in the child's best interest, the court will consider the reasons for the move, the impact of the move on the child and the moving parent, the reasons why the other parent is objecting to the move, and the availability of adequate, alternate custody arrangements if the move is permitted.

If the noncustodial parent does not consent to the move, he/she should file a petition seeking to prohibit the planned move of the custodial parent until after a hearing is held as to whether the move is in the child's best interest.

Where should the action be brought if the noncustodial parent and I live In different states (or counties)?

The action should be brought in the home state of the child. This is the state (or county) in which the child has lived for the preceding six months. There are exceptions:

- If it is in the child's best interest that the action be brought in another state (or county) and the child and at least one parent have significant contacts within that state;

- If the child has been abandoned;

- If it is necessary to protect the child from mistreatment, abuse, or neglect.

If the child was absent from the custodial parent's home state because someone wrongfully removed or kept the child, the custody action can still be brought in the custodial parent's home state.

What constitutes an emergency when seeking immediate custody of a child?

An emergency exists when the child's life, health, or welfare is in immediate danger.

What rights do grandparents have in a custody case?

A grandparent may file a petition for physical and legal custody of a grandchild if the grandparent's relationship with the child began with the consent of the parents or by an order of court. The grandparent must also have assumed the responsibilities of the parent for 12 months or more, or the child must be at risk due to abuse or neglect.

The court may give a grandparent custody where it is not in the child's best interest to be in the custody of either parent, and it is in the child's best interest to be in the custody of the grandparent.

If the parents have been separated for six months or more, if there is a divorce action pending, or if the child has resided with the grandparents for 12 months or more, the grandparents may obtain partial custody or visitation rights. If a parent is deceased, the parents of the deceased parent may also obtain partial custody or visitation rights.

The grandparents' partial custody or visitation must be in the child's best interest and must not interfere with the relationship between the child and the custodial parent.

What are the factors in a custody determination?

The standard in a custody action is the child's best interest. Therefore, all factors and information concerning the child and the parties, which legitimately impact the child, are relevant.

The weight given to each factor in any case will depend upon the unique facts and circumstances of that case.

How much weight or effect is given to the child's preference?

The child's preference is one of many factors. The weight given to the child's preference will depend upon the child's age, competency, and the reasons, communicated by the child, for the child's preference.

Chapter 64

Child Support

About Child Support Enforcement (CSE)

All states and territories run a child support enforcement program, usually in the human services department, department of revenue, or the state Attorney General's office, often with the help of prosecuting attorneys, district attorneys, other law enforcement agencies, and officials of family or domestic relations courts. Native American tribes, too, can operate culturally appropriate child support programs with federal funding. Families seeking government child support services must apply directly through their state/local agency or one of the tribes running the program. Services are available to a parent with custody of a child whose other parent is living outside the home. Services are available automatically for families receiving assistance under the Temporary Assistance for Needy Families (TANF) program.

Services within the CSE include the following:

- Locating noncustodial parents

- Establishing paternity

- Establishing support orders

- Collecting support payments

- Services for noncustodial parents

About This Chapter: Information in this chapter is from the "Office of Child Support Enforcement (OCSE)," January 2009; and "Child Support Enforcement Steps" (undated), both publications of the Administration for Children and Families, U.S. Department of Health and Human Services (www.acf.hhs.gov).

Program Descriptions

Locating Noncustodial Parents

Child support enforcement officials can use information from highly computerized state and federal parent locator services (FPLS) to locate parents and their income and assets.

Establishing Paternity: Legally Identifying A Child's Father

Legally identifying a child's father is called paternity establishment. This is the necessary first step for obtaining an order for child support when a child is born out of wedlock. In addition to providing a legal relationship between a father and child, establishing paternity can provide a child with the following:

- Access to Social Security benefits, pension, and retirement benefits
- Medical insurance and health information
- Important interactions and relationships with both parents

In a disputed case, father, mother, and child can be required to submit to genetic tests. States must have procedures that allow paternity to be established up to the child's 18th birthday. Hospitals must provide fathers the opportunity to acknowledge paternity voluntarily at the time of birth.

Establishing Support Orders

States must have guidelines to determine how much a parent should pay for child support. Child support orders can be established by a court or by an administrative hearing process. Provisions for health insurance coverage must be included in the support order.

Collecting Support

A parent can be required to pay child support by income withholding. Nationally, over 69 percent of child support is paid in this manner. Overdue child support can be collected from the following:

- Federal and state income tax refunds
- Liens placed on property
- Sale of property

It's A Fact!

When past-due child support is owed, the following may occur:

- Unpaid child support can be reported automatically to credit reporting bureaus.
- Driver's, professional, occupational, and recreational licenses can be suspended if the obligated parent is not paying required support.
- The U.S. State Department will deny a passport to someone who owes more than $2,500 in back child support.
- Child support agencies have agreements with financial institutions to freeze and seize accounts of those identified as owing back child support.
- In certain states and under certain circumstances, criminal actions can be taken against chronic delinquent parents who owe large sums of child support.

Source: ACF, HHS, January 2009.

Services For Noncustodial Parents

Noncustodial parents can use the CSE program to establish paternity, establish wage withholding, and request a review of their support orders if circumstances have changed. The federal parent locator service is available through state CSE programs to locate a child who has been hidden in violation of a custody or visitation order.

CSE Highlights

In 2007, 92 percent of child support collections went to families. Welfare recipients now make up just 14 percent of our caseload; the largest group of clients is families who no longer need public assistance, in large part because of child support collections. Preliminary data indicate that, in fiscal year 2007, the following facts were true:

- The program collected nearly $25 billion.
- The total caseload was 15.8 million.
- The FPLS returned employment or address information for over 4.9 million individuals.
- The Multistate Financial Institution Data Match (MSFIDM) program located a quarterly average of 2.6 million accounts containing financial assets owned by over 1.3 million obligors.
- The number of paternities established or acknowledged was 1.7 million.
- The number of new support orders established was 1.2 million.

With the publication of Final Rules and Regulations for Tribal Child Support Enforcement in March 2004, Tribes and Tribal organizations can choose to operate a Title IV-D Tribal Child Support Enforcement Program. Thirty-two comprehensive Tribal programs now can establish paternity, modify and enforce support orders, and locate absent parents. Ten others are receiving federal funding to start new Tribal programs. This will continue to change, however, as more Tribal IV-D programs that operate with start-up funds receive comprehensive status, and as more Tribes receive funds to start new IV-D programs.

In fiscal year (FY) 2007, $3.7 billion in federal funding was provided to states to help defray the costs of the program. Nearly $25 billion was collected at a combined state/federal cost of $5.6 billion; more than $4.73 was collected for each $1 spent. In FY 2007, Tribes across the nation collected and distributed $15.7 million, and forwarded to states an additional $2.2 million, for a total of almost $18 million.

CSE Special Initiatives

The Office of Child Support Enforcement (OCSE) continues to provide technical assistance and training to state CSE agencies through ongoing initiatives such as: the Judicial/Child Support Enforcement Task Force; Hispanic Workgroup; Employer Outreach; and Urban, Interstate, and Interagency initiatives. The project to avoid increasing delinquencies (PAID) began an overarching, national initiative that emphasizes state and local child support activities to increase child support collections as well as prevent and reduce past-due child support obligations. OCSE developed a model automated child support system for use in Tribal IV-D programs, and is working on a regulation that will govern tribal systems development and use of the model system.

Grants provided by the federal government are providing funding to states for programs designed to do the following:

- Provide timely revisions of orders based on ability to pay for categories of persons affected by lowered pay (layoffs, military personnel, prisoners) and related services

- Increase child support enforcement collections and efficiencies through increasing levels of automation or re-engineering of business practices

- Improve child support results through collaboration with other public agencies

- Promote healthy relationships for unwed couples to improve children's financial and medical security

- Improve child support by encouraging parents and CSE agencies to work together for better case management and results

- Expand and improve enforcement and collection tools

Funding

In fiscal year 2009, it is estimated the federal government will provide $3.8 billion to the states for child support enforcement.

Applying For Support

In most states, CSE offices are listed under the human services agency in the local government section of the telephone directory. If there is not a separate listing, the human services agency information operator should be able to give you the number.

Quick Tip

Call your Child Support Enforcement office to learn how to apply for enforcement services and what documents (birth certificates, financial statements, etc.) you should provide.

Source: ACF, HHS, undated.

Steps To Collecting Support

The first step, if a child was born out of wedlock, is to establish paternity—or make a legal determination of who fathered the child. Many men will voluntarily acknowledge paternity. Either parent can request a blood test in contested paternity cases. Your caseworker will help you to establish paternity for your child.

Establishing the obligation is the next step. The fair amount of child support that the non-custodial parent should pay is determined according to state guidelines. Your CSE office will be able to tell you how support award amounts are set in your state. Your CSE office can also request medical support for your child.

The last step is enforcement of the child support order. The CSE office can help with collecting the money due no matter where the noncustodial parent lives.

At any of these steps, the CSE office may need to know where the noncustodial parent is living or where he/she is working. When a parent has disappeared, it is usually possible for the

CSE office to find him/her with the help of state agencies, such as the Department of Motor Vehicles, or the federal parent locator service. Your caseworker can tell you what information is needed to find an absent parent or his/her employer.

The most successful way to collect child support is by direct withholding from the obligated parent's paycheck. Most child support orders require the employer to withhold the money that is ordered for child support and send it to the CSE office. Your Child Support Enforcement office can tell you about this procedure.

Federal and state income tax refunds may be withheld to collect unpaid child support. States also have laws which allow them to use: liens on real and personal property; orders to withhold and deliver property; or seizure and sale of property with the proceeds applied to the support debt. Many states routinely report child support debts to credit bureaus and smart parents are bringing their payments current so that their credit won't be affected.

Chapter 65

Teen Fatherhood Rights And Responsibilities

There is a lot of advice out there for girls who find themselves facing an unwanted or un-expected pregnancy but there is very little information out there for guys. It takes two to make a baby but all too often when the pregnancy is announced the guy gets lost in the confusion. But teen fatherhood is not something to be taken lightly and along with responsibilities to the mother and the child you have rights that you need to know about.

What are your rights as a prospective father?

First and foremost you have the right to know for sure that you are the father. This is not only a right you have but it is a right that the unborn child is entitled to as well. While everyone is mixed up in the emotionally charged circumstances surrounding an unwanted pregnancy it is often overlooked or downplayed that both father and child have a right to know the truth about paternity. Understandably a pregnant girl may be upset when the subject of deoxyribo-nucleic acid (DNA) testing comes up but it is not something you should ever feel guilty about requesting. You are not calling her sexual conduct into question by wanting to know for sure that you are the father. You are not suggesting that she is bad or a liar. You are simply exercising your right to know for sure that you are the father and this is important because fatherhood is a lifelong commitment.

If you are the father you have the right to know your child and to participate in your child's life. You have rights of custody and access. You also have responsibilities. You have the respon-sibility to financially and emotionally care for your child. You have a responsibility to be pres-ent in your child's life and ensure that your child's needs are met. You have the responsibility to ensure that your child is safe and well cared for and is free from harm. You have the responsibility to make decisions that are in the best interest of your child. More on rights and responsibilities later, first let's look at the most important thing every prospective father needs to know about... how to know if he is really the father.

How can you know if you are the father?

There are two ways to determine if you are the father: blood type matching and DNA testing. Blood type matching is the cheapest and simplest test but it does not determine paternity; it only tells you if it is possible that you are the father. If the blood types don't match up there is no possible way you are the father and no other tests are needed. If the blood types do match up it only means that you could be the father and a DNA test will be needed to know for sure.

In order to match blood types you need to know the answers to three questions: what is the father's blood type, what is the mother's blood type, and what is the baby's blood type? A baby's blood type is determined by the blood types of its parents and it is an exact science as to what possible blood type a baby can have based on the types of the parents. It may sound confusing but it is really very simple. The blood type of the baby is determined by a combination of its' parents' blood types. If the baby has a blood type that could not be the result of the combined blood types of both parents then the paternity is usually called into question (since in natural conception maternity is never at issue).

So what is the difference between a positive and a negative blood type match? Rh factor aside (which determines if the blood type is positive + or negative—and is not affected by paternity) a baby will have the same blood type as either its mother or its father or it will have a combined blood type based on the types of both parents. A negative blood type matching happens if a baby does not have the father's or mother's blood type or if the blood type that a baby does have is not a possible combination of the father's and the mother's. A positive blood type matching happens when a baby has the same blood type as the mother, the same blood type as the father, or a blood type that is a combination of the parents' blood types. Table 65.1 shows which blood types are possible based on the combined types of the parents.

Remember in cases of natural conception if the blood types do not match it is because the wrong father has been identified. If the blood types do match up the next step that should be taken is a DNA test as blood type matches only suggest the possibility, not the certainty, that the right father has been identified. DNA testing is much more complicated and expensive but in the end it is worth the investment and many private labs have payment programs available to make access to this test easier. Don't feel bad about wanting a DNA test, as discussed earlier both father and a child have a right to know the truth. The most accurate DNA testing is done using samples from all three parties; mother, identified father, and child, but testing can be done with only samples from the identified father and child. While it is possible to test DNA before a child is born this is much more costly and can pose a risk to the unborn child. For this reason most DNA testing is done after the child is born.

Should you get married?

The question of marriage under these circumstances is a very personal one but it should not be entered into lightly. The pressure to marry when an unwanted pregnancy occurs can be overwhelming but there are important legal ramifications that potential fathers must be aware of. In North America our system of law is based on British Common Law and under this legal structure a child born in wedlock (that is to parents who are legally married at the time of birth) is automatically presumed to belong to the husband. A legal father has the same rights and responsibilities as a biological father. If you marry a girl who claims you fathered her child and later find out that you are not the father it can be difficult and costly, not to mention emotionally devastating, to have your parental rights and responsibilities changed. It may be worth your while to consult with a lawyer near where you live before marrying under these circumstances in order to fully and properly understand the law on this matter where you live.

Table 65.1. Determining Paternity By Blood Type

Parents' Blood Types	You May Be The Father If The Baby Is	You Are Not The Father If The Baby Is
A and A	A, O	B, AB
A and B	A, B, AB, O	All types match
A and AB	A, B, AB	O
A and O	A, O	B, AB
B and B	B, O	A, AB
B and AB	A, B, AB	O
B and O	B, O	A, AB
AB and AB	A, B, AB	O
AB and O	A, B	AB, O
O and O	O	A, B, AB

What about adoption? Can I give up my baby for adoption even if the mother does not want to?

No, you can't force the other parent to give the child up for adoption. You may be able to give up your own parental rights however, depending on the laws where you live. A lawyer in your area can better advise you on the subject of giving up parental rights and obligations and if this is something you want you must seek legal advice.

OK, I'm the father and I'm going to be involved, now what?

If you and the mother can agree on a custody arrangement and on child support it can be as simple as signing an agreement and filing it with the family court in your area. This may or may not require a lawyer. When there is nothing being disputed by either parent then the matter of filing is relatively simple and any associated legal fees are usually minimal. If the two of you can't agree then you will need a lawyer. As a father you have the right to know your child and to be a participant in his or her life. You also have the responsibility to support and care for your child and if you are the noncustodial parent you have the responsibility to pay child support. As touched on earlier you have the responsibility to ensure that your child is free from harm and is well cared for. If you believe that the mother is unable to care for your child or that your child is being harmed in her care then you have a responsibility to do something about it. On the other hand, if a mother believes that you may be bad for the child or put the child in harm's way then she has a responsibility to do something about it. This usually involves going to court to stop or limit access. A lawyer will be needed and depending on where you live you may be able to get legal aid or assistance. Check with your local law society, Attorney General, or other public law office.

It's A Fact!

Parenthood is not an easy thing and it should never be entered into lightly. No matter what the circumstances surrounding conception when you become a parent you are a parent for the rest of your life. Fathers are no less important than mothers and their obligations to their child are no less than those of a mother. Just because biology has made it that mothers carry the child in their body this does not mean that the mother is the most important parent. Both parents have important roles to play in the life of their child. While having a child while you're still a kid yourself is less than ideal this does not make you any less a parent. Once you know a child is yours it changes your life forever no matter how old, or young, you are.

Part Eight
If You Need More Information

Chapter 66

Directory Of Teen Pregnancy Resources

Information About Sexual Health, Pregnancy, And Birth

Advocates for Youth

2000 M Street NW, Suite 750
Washington, DC 20036
Phone: 202-419-3420
Fax: 202-419-1448
Website:
http://www.advocatesforyouth.org

American College of Nurse-Midwives (ACNM)

8403 Colesville Road, Suite 1550
Silver Spring, MD 20910
Phone: 240-485-1800
Fax: 240-485-1818
Website: http://www.midwife.org

American College of Obstetricians and Gynecologists (ACOG)

409 12th Street SW
P.O. Box 96920
Washington, DC 20090-6920
Phone: 202-638-5577
Website: http://www.acog.org
E-mail: resources@acog.org

American Pregnancy Association

1425 Greenway Drive, Suite 440
Irving, TX 75038
Toll-Free: 800-672-2296
Phone: 972-550-0140
Fax: 972-550-0800
Website: http://www.americanpregnancy.org
E-mail: Questions@AmericanPregnancy.org

About This Chapter: Information in this chapter was compiled from many sources deemed reliable; inclusion does not constitute endorsement. All contact information was verified and updated in September 2011.

American Social Health Association (ASHA)

P.O. Box 13827
Research Triangle Park, NC 27709
Phone: 919-361-8400
Fax: 919-361-8425
Website: http://www.ashastd.org
E-mail: info@ashastd.org
Teen-Oriented Website:
http://www.iwannaknow.org

Campaign for Our Children, Inc. (CFOC)

One North Charles Street, 11th Floor
Baltimore, MD 21201
Phone: 410-576-9015
Fax: 410-752-7075
Website: http://www.cfoc.org

Childbirth Connection

260 Madison, 8th Floor
New York, NY 10016
Phone: 212-777-5000
Fax: 212-777-9320
Website:
http://www.childbirthconnection.org

Child Care Aware

1515 North Courthouse Road, 11th Floor
Arlington, VA 22201
Toll-Free: 800-424-2246
Toll-Free TTY: 866-278-9428
Fax: 703-341-4101
Website: http://www.childcareaware.org

Child Welfare Information Gateway

Children's Bureau/ACYF
1250 Maryland Avenue SW, Eighth Floor
Washington, DC 20024
Toll-Free: 800-394-3366
Phone: 703-385-7565
Fax: 703-385-3206
Website: http://www.childwelfare.gov
E-mail: info@childwelfare.gov

Focus Adolescent Services

P.O. Box 4514
Salisbury, MD 21803
Toll-Free: 877-362-8727
Phone: 410-341-4216
Website: http://www.focusas.com
E-mail: help@focusas.com

Guttmacher Institute

125 Maiden Lane, 7th Floor
New York, NY 10038
Toll-Free: 800-355-0244
Phone: 212-248-1111
Fax: 212-248-1951
Website: http://www.guttmacher.org
E-mail: info@guttmacher.org

Lamaze International

2025 M Street NW, Suite 800
Washington, DC 20036-3309
Toll-Free: 800-368-4404
Phone: 202-367-1128
Fax: 202-367-2128
Website: http://www.lamaze.org
E-mail: info@lamaze.org

Life in the Fast Lane

Website: http://www.teenageparent.org

March of Dimes

Pregnancy and Newborn Health Service
Center
1275 Mamaroneck Avenue
White Plains, NY 10605
Phone: (914) 997-4488
Website: http://www.marchofdimes.com/
pnhec/pnhec.asp

Black Women's Health Imperative

Formerly known as National Black
Women's Health Project
1726 M Street NW, Suite 300
Washington, DC 20036
Phone: 202-548-4000
Fax: 203-543-9743
Website:
http://www.blackwomenshealth.org

The National Campaign to Prevent Teen and Unplanned Pregnancy

1776 Massachusetts Avenue NW
Suite 200
Washington, DC 20036
Phone: 202-478-8500
Fax: 202-478-8588
Website: http://www.teenpregnancy.org
Teen Website: http://stayteen.org/
E-mail: campaign@teenpregnancy.org

National Domestic Violence Hotline

P.O. Box 161810
Austin, TX 78716
Toll-Free: 800-799-SAFE (7233)
Toll-Free TTY: 800-787-3224
Phone: 512-794-1133
Website: http://www.thehotline.org/

Eunice Kennedy Shriver

National Institute of Child Health and
Human Development (NICHD)
Information Resource Center
P.O. Box 3006
Rockville, MD 20847
Toll-Free: 800-370-2943
Toll-Free TTY: 888-320-6942
Toll-Free Fax: 866-760-5947
Website: http://www.nichd.nih.gov
E-mail: NICHDInformationResource
Center@mail.nih.gov

Health Resources and Services Administration (HRSA)

Maternal and Child Health
HRSA Information Center
P.O. Box 2910
Merrifield, VA 22116
Toll-Free: 888-ASK-HRSA
(888- 275-4772)
Toll-Free TTY/TTD: 877-4TY-HRSA
(877-489-4772)
Toll-Free: 800-311-BABY
(800-311-2229) for Prenatal Services
Fax: 703-821-2098
Website: http://mchb.hrsa.gov/
E-mail: ask@hrsa.gov

National Sexual Assault Hotline

Toll-Free: 800-656-HOPE
(800-656-4673)

Womenshealth.gov

U.S. Department of Health and Human Services
8270 Willow Oaks Corporate Drive
Suite 101
Fairfax, VA 22031
Toll-Free: 800-994-9662
Toll-Free TDD: 888-220-5446
Phone: 202-690-7650
Fax: 202-205-2631
Website: http://www.womenshealth.gov/
Pregnancy

Planned Parenthood Federation of America

434 West 33rd Street
New York, NY 10001
Toll-Free: 800-230-PLAN
(800-230-7526)
Phone: 212-541-7800
Fax: 212-245-1845
Website:
http://www.plannedparenthood.org/

Preeclampsia Foundation

6767 North Wickham Road, Suite 400
Melbourne, FL 32940
Toll-Free: 800-665-9341
Phone: 321-421-6957
Fax: 321-821-0450
Website: http://www.preeclampsia.org/
E-mail: info@preeclampsia.org

Sexuality Information and Education Council of the United States (SIECUS)

90 John Street, Suite 402
New York, NY 10038
Phone: 212-819-9770
Fax: 212-819-9776
Website: http://www.siecus.org
E-mail: siecus@siecus.org

U.S. Department of Health and Human Services (HHS)

Administration for Children and Families
370 L'Enfant Promenade SW
Washington, DC 20447
Website: http://www.acf.hhs.gov

Breastfeeding and Postpartum Support

International Lactation Consultant Association (ILCA)

2501 Aerial Center Parkway, Suite 103
Morrisville, NC 27560
Toll-Free: 888-ILCA-IS-U
(888-452-2478)
Phone: 919-861-5577
Fax: 919-459-2075
Website: www.ilca.org
E-mail: info@ilca.org

La Leche League International (LLLI)

957 North Plum Grove Road
Schaumburg, IL 60173
Toll-Free: 800-LALECHE
(800-525-3243)
Phone: 847-519-7730
Fax: 847-969-0460
Website: www.lalecheleague.org

Nursing Mothers Counsel (NMC)

P.O. Box 5024
San Mateo, CA 94402-0024
Phone: 650-327-MILK (650-327-6455)
Website: www.nursingmothers.org
E-mail: info@nursingmothers.org

Postpartum Education for Parents (PEP)

P.O. Box 261
Santa Barbara, CA 93116
Phone: 805-564-3888 (24–hour service)
Website: www.sbpep.org
E-mail: pepboard@sbpep.org

Chapter 67

Directory Of Assistance Resources For Low-Income Pregnant Women

American Public Human Services Association (APHSA)

1133 19th Street NW, Suite 400
Washington, DC 20036
Phone: 202-682-0100
Fax: 202-289-6555
Website: http://www.aphsa.org

Center for Health Care Strategies, Inc. (CHCS)

200 American Metro Boulevard, Suite 119
Hamilton, NJ 08619
Phone: 609-528-8400
Fax: 609-586-3679
Website: http://www.chcs.org
E-mail: mail@chcs.org

Centers for Medicare and Medicaid Services (CMS)

7500 Security Boulevard
Baltimore, MD 21244-1850
Toll-Free: 877-267-2323
Toll-Free TTY: 866-226-1819
Phone: 410-786-3000
TTY: 410-786-0727
Website: http://www.cms.gov/

Children's Health Insurance Program (CHIP)

7500 Security Boulevard
Baltimore, MD 21244
Phone: 1-877-KIDS-NOW
(1-877-543-7669)
Website:
https://www.cms.gov/home/chip.asp

About This Chapter: Information in this chapter was compiled from many sources deemed reliable; inclusion does not constitute endorsement. All contact information was verified and updated in September 2011.

National Academy for State Health Policy

10 Free Street, Second Floor
Portland, ME 04101
Phone: 207-874-6524
Fax: 207-874-6527
Website: http://www.nashp.org
E-mail: info@nashp.org

National Advocates for Pregnant Women (NAPW)

15 West 36th Street, Suite 901
New York, NY 10018-7910
Phone: 212-255-9252
Fax: 212-255-9253
Website: http://advocatesforpregnant
women.org
E-mail:
info@advocatesforpregnantwomen.org

National Association of Public Hospitals and Health Systems (NAPH)

1301 Pennsylvania Avenue NW, Suite 950
Washington, DC 20004
Phone: 202-585-0100
Fax: 202-585-0101
Website: http://www.naph.org
E-mail: info@naph.org

National Coalition on Health Care (NCHC)

1200 G Street NW, Suite 810
Washington, DC 20005
Phone: 202-638-7151
Fax: 202-638-7166
Website: http://www.nchc.org

National Health Law Program (NHelp)

3701 Wilshire Boulevard, Suite 750
Los Angeles, CA 90010
Phone: 310-204-6010
Fax: 310-368-0774
Website: http://www.healthlaw.org
E-mail: nhelp@healthlaw.org

National Health Policy Forum

2131 K Street NW, Suite 500
Washington DC 20037
Phone: 202-872-1390
Fax: 202-862-9837
Website: http://www.nhpf.org
E-mail: nhpf@gwu.edu

National Rural Health Association (NRHA)

521 East 63rd Street
Kansas City, MO 64110-3329
Phone: 816-756-3140
Fax: 816-756-3144
Website: http://www.nrharural.org
E-mail: mail@NRHArural.org

Office of Rural Health Policy

Health Resources and Services
Administration (HRSA)
5600 Fishers Lane, 10B-45
Rockville, MD 20857
Phone: 301-443-0835
Fax: 301-443-2803
Website: http://www.hrsa.gov/ruralhealth/
E-mail: orthpwebsite@hrsa.gov

Robert Wood Johnson Foundation

Route 1 and College Road East
P.O. Box 2316
Princeton, NJ 08543
Toll-Free: 877-843-RWJF
(877-843-7953)
Website: http://www.rwjf.org

Second Chance Homes

U.S. Department of Housing and Urban
Development (HUD)
451 7th Street SW
Washington, DC 20410
Phone: 202-708-1112
TTY: 202-708-1455
Website: http://portal.hud.gov/hudportal
/HUD?src=/program_offices/public
_indian_housing/other/sch

State Coverage Initiatives (SCI)

Academy Health
1150 17th Street NW, Suite 600
Washington, DC 20036
Phone: 202-292-6731
Fax: 202-292-6800
Website: http://www.statecoverage.org/
E-mail: sci@academyhealth.org

Temporary Assistance for Needy Families (TANF)

U.S. Department of Health and Human
Services
Administration for Children and Families
370 L'Enfant Promenade, SW
Washington, D.C. 20447
Phone: 202-724-5506
Website: http://www.acf.hhs.gov/
programs/ofa/tanf/about.html

Urban Institute

2100 M Street NW
Washington, DC 20037
Phone: 202-833-7200
Website: http://www.urban.org

Women, Infants, and Children (WIC)

Supplemental Food Programs Division
Food and Nutrition Service—USDA
3101 Park Center Drive, Room 520
Alexandria, VA 22302
Phone: 703-305-2746
Fax: 703-305-2196
Website: http://www.fns.usda.gov/wic
Directory of Regional WIC Offices:
http://www.fns.usda.gov/wic/Contacts/
fnsoffices.htm
E-mail: wichq-web@fns.usda.gov

Chapter 68

Directory Of Education Resources For Teen Parents

American Council on Education (ACE)

One Dupont Circle NW
Washington, DC 20036-1193
Phone: 202-939-9300
Website: http://www.acenet.edu
GED Testing Service: http://www.acenet
.edu/AM/Template.cfm?Section=GEDTS
E-mail: comments@ace.nche.edu

Job Corps

U.S. Department of Labor
200 Constitution Avenue NW
Suite N4463
Washington, DC 20210
Toll-Free: 800-773-JOBS (800-773-5627)
Toll-Free TTY: 877-889-5627
Phone: 202-693-3000
Fax: 202-693-2767
Website: http://jobcorps.dol.gov
E-mail: national_office@jobcorps.gov

U.S. Department of Education (ED)

400 Maryland Avenue SW
Washington, DC 20202
Toll Free: 800-USA-LEARN
(800-872-5327)
Toll-Free TTY: 800-437-0833
Phone: 202-401-2000
Fax: 202-401-0689
Website: http://www.ed.gov

About This Chapter: Information in this chapter was compiled from many sources deemed reliable; inclusion does not constitute endorsement. All contact information was verified and updated in September 2011.

Online Directories For State-Specific Help

American Association Of Community Colleges

Assists you in locating a community college that can serve your continuing education needs.
Website: http://www.aacc.nche.edu/Pages/default.aspx

State Coordinator Of Education For Homeless Children And Youth

Ensures that all homeless children and youth have equal access to the same free, appropriate public education, including public preschool education, provided to other children and youth; develops, reviews, and revises policies to remove barriers to the enrollment, attendance, and success in school of homeless children and youth; provides them with opportunities to meet the same challenging state content and state student performance standards to which all students are held.
Website: http://wdcrobcolp01.ed.gov/Programs/EROD/org_list.cfm?category_cd=SHC

State Director Of Adult Education

Provides students with opportunities to develop skills needed to qualify for further education, job training, and better employment.
Website: http://wdcrobcolp01.ed.gov/Programs/EROD/org_list.cfm?category_cd=DAE

State Tech Prep Coordinator

Prepares students for a highly skilled, technical occupation that allows either direct entry into the workplace as a qualified technician or further education leading to baccalaureate and advanced degrees. Tech Prep is a four-year sequence of study from the 11th grade through two years of post secondary occupation education culminating in a certificate or associate degree.
Website: http://wdcrobcolp01.ed.gov/Programs/EROD/org_list.cfm?category_ID=TPC

Financial Aid Information For Post-Secondary Education

College Board Scholarship Search

National Office
45 Columbus Avenue
New York, NY 10023-6917
Toll-Free: 866-630-9305
Phone: 212-713-8000
Website: http://apps.collegeboard.com/cbsearch_ss/welcome.jsp

Civil Rights of Pregnant and Parenting Teens in California Schools

California Women's Law Center
URL: http://www.cwlc.org/m/2011/02/policy_brief_civil_rights_ppt.pdf

FastWeb

FastWeb, LLC
444 North Michigan Avenue, Suite 600
Chicago, IL 60611
Website: http://www.fastweb.com
E-mail: info@fastweb.com

Federal Student Aid

Toll-Free: 800-4-FED-AID
(800-433-3243)
Toll-Free TTY: 800-730-8913
Phone: 319-337-5665
Website: http://studentaid.ed.gov

FinAid

FinAid Page, LLC
P.O. Box 2056
Cranberry Township, PA 16066-1056
Phone: 724-538-4500
Fax: 724-538-4502
Website: http://www.finaid.org
E-mail: questions@finaid.org

Free Application for Federal Student Aid (FAFSA)

Toll-Free: 800-4-FED-AID
(800-433-3243)
Toll-Free TTY: 800-730-8913
Phone: 319-337-5665
Website: http://www.fafsa.ed.gov

National Association of Student Financial Aid Administrators (NASFAA)

1101 Connecticut Avenue NW, Suite 1100
Washington, DC 20036-4303
Phone: 202-785-0453
Fax: 202-785-1487
Website: http://www.nasfaa.org

SallieMae

P.O. Box 9532
Wilkes-Barre, PA 18773-9532
Toll-Free: 888-2-SALLIE
(888-272-5543)
Toll-Free TDD: 888-TDD-SLMA
(888-833-7562)
Phone: 317-570-7397
Toll-Free Fax: 800-848-1949
Website: http://www.salliemae.com

Additional Reading About Education For Teen Parents

Career Education for Teen Parents

Eric Digest
URL: http://www.ericdigests.org/1995-2/teen.htm

Helping the Education System Work for Teen Parents and Their Children

Center for Assessment and Policy Development
URL: http://www.capd.org/pubfiles/pub-1999-10-06.pdf

Rights of Pregnant and Parenting Teens

New York Civil Liberties Union
URL: http://www.nyclu.org/publications/booklet-rights-of-pregnant-and-parenting-teens-2006

School-Based and School-Linked Programs for Pregnant and Parenting Teens and Their Children

U.S. Department of Education
URL: http://www.ed.gov/PDFDocs/teenparent.pdf

Schools Failing to Accommodate Teens Who Are Pregnant or New Mothers

University of Illinois at Urbana-Champaign
URL: http://www.news.uiuc.edu/NEWS/04/0423pregnant.html

Index

Index

Page numbers that appear in *Italics* refer to tables or illustrations. Page numbers that have a small 'n' after the page number refer to information shown as Notes at the beginning of each chapter. Page numbers that appear in **Bold** refer to information contained in boxes on that page (except Notes information at the beginning of each chapter).

A

alcohol use, *continued*
    overview 131–35
    pregnancy 70
    recommendations **134**
allergies, overview 201–4
allergy shots, pregnancy 204
American Association of Community
    Colleges, website address 376
American College of Allergy, Asthma,
    and Immunology (ACAAI), asthma
    management publication 201n
American College of Nurse-Midwives (ACNM),
    contact information 365
American College of Obstetricians and
    Gynecologists (ACOG), contact information 365
American Council on Education (ACE),
    contact information 375
American Pregnancy Association
    contact information 365
    publications
        birth plans 247n
        caffeine use 141n
        eating disorders 105n
        pregnancy symptoms 41n
American Public Human Services Association
    (APHSA), contact information 371
American Social Health Association (ASHA),
    contact information 366
amniocentesis
    described 79–80
    genetic testing 173
amniotic fluid, described 257, **258**
amphetamines, pregnancy 146–47
anemia
    age factor 167
    overview 185–88
    pregnancy complications 179
"Anemia" (March of Dimes Birth Defects
    Foundation) 185n
Apgar score
    described 270
    medical care **271**
areola darkening, pregnancy 44
"Are You Pregnant and Thinking About Adoption?"
    (Child Welfare Information Gateway) 55n

ARND *see* alcohol related
    neurodevelopmental disorders
arsenic, health risks 156
ART *see* assisted reproductive technology
Asian/Pacific Islanders, birth rates 9–11
assisted reproductive technology (ART),
    multiple births 213
asthma
    overview 201–4
    pregnancy complications 177
    secondhand smoke 138
"Available Resources - Second Chance
    Homes" (HUD) 313n
AZT *see* zidovudine

B

baby blues, described 116
baby-friendly hospitals, described **76**
baby needs *see* layette
babysitters
    versus child care programs 341
    safety considerations **341**
"Baby's Layette" (Office on Women's Health) 235n
backaches
    pregnancy 42, 91
    sleep problems 110
bacterial vaginosis, described 181
barrier methods, birth control 29–30
"Bathing an Infant" (A.D.A.M., Inc.) 287n
biophysical profile (BPP), described 80
birth centers
    epidurals **77**
    labor and delivery 76–77, 253–56
birth control methods, overview 29–34
"Birth Control Methods: Frequently Asked
    Questions" (DHHS) 29n
birth defects
    caffeine 141–42
    causes **128**
    fetal alcohol syndrome 132
    folic acid 83–85
    genetic testing 174
    tobacco use 138
    vitamins 124–25

F

fallopian tubes, ectopic pregnancy 219–20

false labor, described 258

family child care home programs,
    described 337

family issues
    breastfeeding 280
    child custody 347–51
    child support 353–58
    emancipation 299–303
    first trip home 284–85
    housing options 305–8

FAS *see* fetal alcohol syndrome

FASD *see* fetal alcohol spectrum disorders

FastWeb, contact information 377

fathers
    adoptions 55–57
    alcohol use 135
    breastfeeding 280
    overview 359–62

fatigue, pregnancy 42, 92–93

FDA *see* US Food and Drug Administration

federal parent locator services (FPLS),
    described 354

Federal Student Aid, contact information 377

fee for service insurance, described 324

female condom, described 30

fertility, eating disorders 105

fetal alcohol spectrum disorders (FASD),
    overview 131–35

fetal alcohol syndrome (FAS), described 132

fetal monitoring
    described 78
    maternal asthma 202

fetus, described **232**

FinAid, contact information 377

financial considerations
    breastfeeding 276, 277
    child care programs 338–39, 343–46
    child support 355–56
    prenatal care 82
    WIC program 332

"Finding Help Paying for Child Care"
    (NACCRRA) 343n

first aid
    babysitters **341**
    CPR 242–44

first trimester
    described 87–88
    fetal development 231–32
    maternal asthma 202
    screening test 80

"Fit for Two: Tips for Pregnancy" (NIDDK) 97n

flu-like symptoms, treatment **182**

flu shot
    described 181
    pregnancy 204

Focus Adolescent Services,
    contact information 366

folate, described 85

folic acid, overview 83–85

"Folic Acid Questions and Answers" (CDC) 83n

Food and Drug Administration (FDA)
    see US Food and Drug Administration

Food and Nutrition Service (FNS)
    described **330**
    website address **332**

food cravings, pregnancy 44

food poisoning, pregnancy **100, 101**

formula
    versus breastmilk 275
    WIC rebates 332

formula feeding, described **276**

fraternal twins, described 214

Free Application for Federal Student
    Aid (FAFSA), contact information 377

free clinics, health care 326

frequent urination, pregnancy 43, 96

G

galactosemia, newborn screening 272

general equivalency diploma (GED)
    described 295–96
    second chance homes 313–14

"Genetic Testing" (Nemours Foundation) 173n

genetic testing, overview 173–75

Georgetown University, Maternal and Child
    Health Library, contact information **163**